Journal of **Vascular Research**

General Information

Publication data: 'Journal of Vascular Research' is published 6 times a year. Volume 41 with 6 issues appears in 2004.

Subscription rates: Subscriptions run for a full calendar year. Prices are given per year.

Personal subscription:

Print or Online	Print/Online combined
CHF 94.–	CHF 135.–
EUR 67.–	EUR 97.–
USD 72.00	USD 105.00
postage and handling	(added to print and print/online)
CHF 31.80 Europe,	CHF 47.10 Overseas
EUR 22.80	
USD 31.80	

Institutional subscription:

Print or Online	Print/Online combined
CHF 1128.–	CHF 1218.–
EUR 836.–	EUR 902.–
USD 902.00	USD 974.00
postage and handling	(added to print and print/online)
CHF 39.60 Europe,	CHF 58.80 Overseas
EUR 28.50	
USD 39.60	

Airmail surcharge: CHF 39.60 / USD 33.00

Microforms: Please direct all enquiries and orders to:
University Microfilms Inc.
300 North Zeeb Road, P.O. Box 1346
Ann Arbor, MI 48106-1346 (USA)

Subscription orders: Orders can be placed at agencies, bookstores, directly with the Publisher
S. Karger AG, P.O. Box
CH–4009 Basel (Switzerland)
or with any of the following distributors:
Deutschland: S. Karger GmbH, Postfach
D–79095 Freiburg
France: Librairie Luginbühl
36, bd de Latour-Maubourg
F–75007 Paris
Great Britain, Ireland: S. Karger AG
4 Rickett Street
London SW6 1RU, UK
USA: S. Karger Publishers, Inc.
26 West Avon Road, P.O. Box 529
Farmington, CT 06085, USA
India, Bangladesh, Sri Lanka:
Panther Publishers Private Ltd.
33, First Main
Koramangala First Block
Bangalore 560 034, India
Japan: Karger Japan, Inc.
Yushima S Bld. 3F
4-2-3, Yushima, Bunkyo-ku
Tokyo 113-0034, Japan

Change of address: Both old and new address should be sent to the subscription source.

Single issues and back volumes: Information can be obtained through the Publisher.

Advertising: Correspondence and rate requests should be addressed to the Publisher.

Bibliographic indices: This journal is regularly listed in bibliographic services, including *Current Contents*® and Index Medicus/MEDLINE.

Copying: This journal has been registered with the Copyright Clearance Center (CCC), as indicated by the code appearing on the first page of each article. For readers in the US, this code signals consent for copying of articles for personal or internal use, or for the personal or internal use of specific clients, provided that the stated fee is paid per copy directly to
Copyright Clearance Center Inc.
222 Rosewood Drive
Danvers, MA 01923 (USA)
A copy of the first page of the article must accompany payment. Consent does not extend to copying for general distribution, for promotion, for creating new works, or for resale. In these cases, specific written permission must be obtained from the copyright owner,
S. Karger AG,
P.O. Box, CH–4009 Basel (Switzerland).

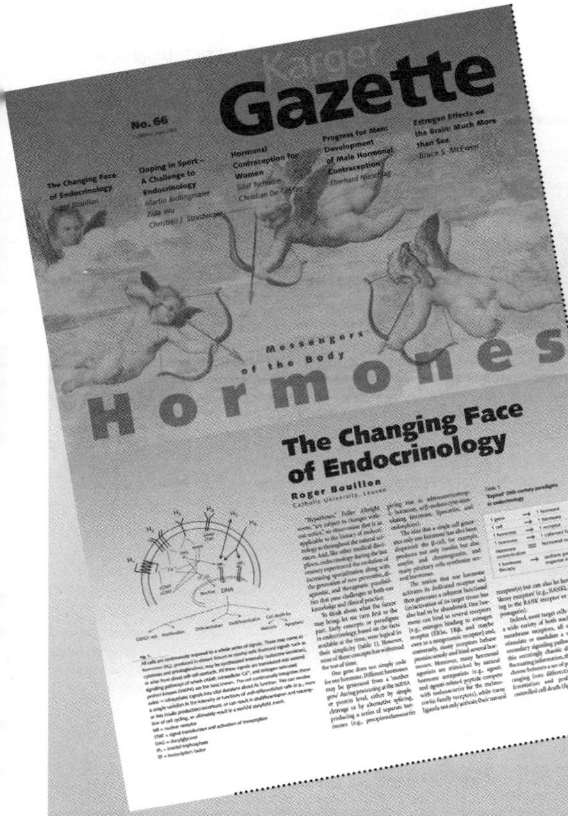

Not just for specialists

The biomedical themes of the *Karger Gazette* are topical, urgent, exciting. Its articles, written by experts from all over the world, provide a wide audience with the basic issues, new findings and controversies in a lively and readable style. Alongside invited contributions, each number carries attractively presented support material, such as informative graphics, historical summaries, interviews, and portraits of individuals and institutions. The *Karger Gazette* appears once a year. And what's more – it's free. To see behind the cover, please write, fax or e-mail us, and we'll start your subscription with the latest issue.

Online: www.karger.com/gazette

KARGER

S. Karger AG
Karger Gazette
P.O. Box
CH–4009 Basel (Switzerland)
Fax +41 61 306 12 34
E-Mail gazette@karger.ch
www.karger.com

KI 03245

KARGER

Fax +41 61 306 12 34
E-Mail karger@karger.ch
www.karger.com

© 2004 S. Karger AG, Basel

The Journal Home Page is available at:
www.karger.com/jvr

A comprehensive analysis of the most recent findings

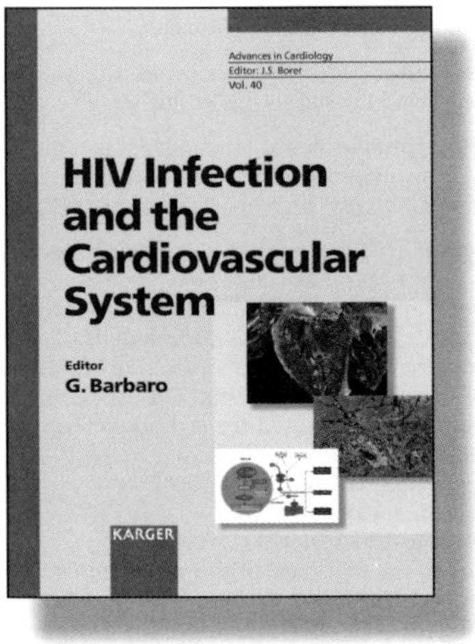

HIV Infection and the Cardiovascular System

Editor
Giuseppe Barbaro

Cardiovascular System; Internal Medicine; AIDS, Infectious Diseases, Metabolic Diseases, Pharmacology

Past studies revealed that HIV infection may implicate diverse cardiac diseases such as cardiomyopathy, coronary heart disease, cardiac neoplasms, endocarditis or pericarditis. In addition, it was found that highly active antiretroviral therapy (HAART) often causes – as an adverse effect – a metabolic syndrome characterized by lipodystrophy/lipoatrophy, dyslipidemia and insulin resistance, leading to an increase in coronary artery disease and stroke.
This book focuses on the most recent findings in HIV-associated heart disease and HAART-associated metabolic and cardiovascular complications. In a first part, the epidemiology, pathogenesis and molecular biology of HIV-associated cardiovascular disease, pulmonary hypertension, lipodystrophy and HAART-associated metabolic syndrome are reviewed. The second part offers clinical and therapeutic insights into HIV/HAART-associated atherosclerosis, coronary heart disease, stroke, vasculitic syndromes, and pulmonary hypertension. Besides, cardiovascular complications in HIV-infected children, cardiac surgery in HIV-infected patients, and the prevention and management of HAART-associated cardiovascular complications are points under discussion. Finally, the interaction between HAART and drugs commonly used to treat cardiovascular disease is carefully analyzed.
HIV Infection and the Cardiovascular System presents state-of-the-art findings of basic and clinical scientists and is a valuable reference for specialists in cardiology and internal medicine as well as for infectiologists.

KI 03253

Contents

Foreword: ***Fiala, M.***
HAART and Cardiology – Current Controversies and Consequences: ***Hoffmann, C.; Jaeger, H.***

Epidemiology, Pathogenesis and Molecular Biology
Evolution of the Involvement of the Cardiovascular System in HIV Infection: ***Barbaro, G.***
Cardiovascular Pathology in AIDS: ***Klatt, E.C.***
Pathogenesis of HIV-Associated Cardiovascular Disease: ***Barbaro, G.***
The Pathogenesis of HIV-Associated Pulmonary Hypertension: ***Klings, E.S.; Farber, H.W.***
Pathogenesis of the HAART-Associated Metabolic Syndrome: ***Behrens, G.M.N.; Stoll, M.; Schmidt, R.E.***
HIV-Associated Lipodystrophy: Pathogenesis and Clinical Features: ***Barbaro, G.***

Clinical and Therapeutic Insights
Assessment of Autonomic and Cardiovascular Function in HIV Disease: ***Brownley, K.A.; Hurwitz, B.E.***
Atherosclerosis and HIV Infection: Diagnosis and Treatment: ***Mooser, V.***
Coronary Heart Disease in HIV-Infected Individuals: ***Vittecoq, D.; Escaut, L.; Merad, M.; Teicher, E.; Monsuez, J.J., Chironi, G.***
Coronary Artery Disease and Stroke in HIV-Infected Patients: Prevention and Pharmacological Therapy: ***Boccara, F.; Cohen, A.***
Vasculitic Syndromes in HIV-Infected Patients: ***Barbaro, G.***
HIV-Associated Pulmonary Hypertension: Diagnosis and Treatment: ***Burkart, K.M.; Farber, H.W.***
HIV-Associated Cardiovascular Complication in HIV-Infected Children: ***Bonnet, D.***
Cardiac Surgery in the Patient with Human Immunodeficiency Virus: ***Frater, R.W.M.; Comacho, M.; Frymus, M.; Soeiro, R.; Zingman, B.S.***
Guidelines for the Prevention and Management of Cardiovascular Complications in HIV-Infected Patients Receiving HAART: The Pavia Consensus Statement: ***Barbaro, G.***

Appendix
Interactions between Antiretroviral Agents and Drugs Commonly Used to Treat Cardiovascular Diseases According to the Pavia Consensus Statement: ***Barbaro, G.***

Author Index
Subject Index

www.karger.com/adcar

Advances in Cardiology, Vol. 40
Series Editor: Borer, J.S. (New York, N.Y.)
ISSN 0065–2326

HIV Infection and the Cardiovascular System
Editor: Barbaro, G. (Rome)
VIII + 248 p., 24 fig., 13 in color, 25 tab., hard cover, 2003
CHF 190.– / EUR 135.50 / USD 165.25
Prices subject to change
EUR price for Germany, USD price for USA only
ISBN 3–8055–7606–4

KARGER

Order Form

Please send: ____ copy/ies
Postage and handling free with prepayment

Payment:
☐ Check enclosed ☐ Please bill me

Please charge to my credit card
☐ American Express ☐ Diners ☐ Eurocard
☐ MasterCard ☐ Visa

Card No.: ____________

Exp. date: ____________

Orders may be placed with any bookshop, subscription agency, directly with the publisher or through a Karger distributor.

Fax: +41 61 306 12 34
S. Karger AG, P.O. Box, CH–4009 Basel (Switzerland)
E-Mail orders@karger.ch, **www.karger.com**

Name/Address: ____________

Date: ____________

Signature: ____________

Official Journal of the European Society for Microcirculation

Journal of Vascular Research

Founded 1964 as 'Angiologica' by M. Comèl and L. Laszt (1964–1973)
continued as 'Blood Vessels' by J.A. Bevan (1974–1991)
continued as 'Journal of Vascular Research' by M.J. Mulvany (1991–2002)

Incorporating International Journal of Microcirculation, Clinical and Experimental, founded 1980 by the European Society for Microcirculation

Main Editor

U. Pohl, Munich

Co-Editor

G.A. Meininger, College Station, Tex.

Consulting Editors

J.G.R. DeMey, Maastricht
I. Fleming, Frankfurt/Main
M.D. Menger, Homburg/Saar
J.D. Pearson, London
M. Ziche, Siena

Editorial Assistants

T. Crow, College Station, Tex.
E. Aralikatti, Munich

Editorial Board

E. van Bavel, Amsterdam
B.C. Berk, Rochester, N.Y.
A. Bobik, Melbourne
R. Busse, Frankfurt/Main
J. Campbell, Brisbane
M.J.A.P. Daemen, Maastricht
P.F. Davies, Philadelphia, Pa.
M.J. Davis, College Station, Tex.
P.E. DiCorleto, Cleveland, Ohio
C.J. Garland, Bath
M. Gassmann, Zürich
M. Gollasch, Berlin
S.L. Gonias, Charlottesville, Va.
A.S. Greene, Milwaukee, Wisc.
H. Haller, Hannover
D.G. Harrison, Atlanta, Ga.
A.M. Heagerty, Manchester
P. Hellstrand, Lund
G. Heusch, Essen
V.W. van Hinsbergh, Leiden
A.D. Hughes, London
V.H. Huxley, Columbia, Mo.
W.F. Jackson, Kalamazoo, Mich.
I. Laher, Vancouver
B.L. Langille, Toronto
P. Libby, Boston, Mass.
T.M. Lincoln, Birmingham, Ala.
L. Lindbom, Stockholm
J. Linden, Charlottesville, Va.
J. Lopez-Barneo, Sevilla
M.W. Majesky, Houston, Tex.
J.M. Marshall, Birmingham
J.C. McGrath, Glasgow
A.C. Newby, Bristol
H. Nilsson, Aarhus
R.L. Prewitt, Norfolk, Va.
A.R. Pries, Berlin
T.J. Resink, Basel
E.L. Schiffrin, Montréal
G.W. Schmid-Schönbein, La Jolla, Calif.
S.M. Schwartz, Seattle, Wash.
S.S. Segal, New Haven, Conn.
W.C. Sessa, New Haven, Conn.
A.C. Shore, Exeter
U. Simonsen, Aarhus
T.C. Skalak, Charlottesville, Va.
D.W. Slaaf, Maastricht
N.B. Standen, Leicester
H.A.J. Struijker-Boudier, Maastricht
A. Tedgui, Paris
J.E. Tooke, Exeter
E. Vicaut, Paris
R.M. Wadsworth, Glasgow

KARGER

Printed in Switzerland
on acid-free paper by
Reinhardt Druck, Basel

Appears bimonthly:
1 volume per year
(6 issues)

Journal of Vascular Research

Guidelines for Authors

The Journal of Vascular Research publishes manuscripts of scientific distinction in the vascular, microvascular and lymphatic fields, as regards biology, physiology and pathophysiology, with an emphasis on mechanisms. The scope of the journal covers a broad spectrum of research, including structure, function, hemodynamics, mechanics, pharmacology, cell signalling, intercellular communication, growth and differentiation. Papers employing cellular, biophysical, molecular and intravital microscopic as well as more classical techniques are welcome. Clinical approaches (especially in the field of microcirculation) will be readily considered only if they provide new insights into the origin or rational therapy of diseases. Manuscripts may be in the form of research papers, reviews, short communications, letters to the editor, commentaries and new methods in vascular research. In all cases, the criteria for acceptance are based on completeness, novelty and scientific excellence.

Submission

Only original papers written in English are considered. Research papers and reviews should not normally be more than 10 printed pages in length including illustrations and references (approximately 6,460 characters, spaces included per printed page). Authors wishing to submit a Review should contact the Editors in advance. Short communications should not exceed 3 printed pages.

Manuscripts to the *Journal of Vascular Research* can now be submitted online! Detailed online submission instructions with a link to the submission website are at **http://oper.karger.com/jvr/**. Before submitting your manuscript, you are encouraged to review the detailed guidelines at **www.karger.com/jvr_guidelines** for specific directions as how to get a manuscript ready for submission. Should you have any problems with your submission or feel the need to submit the paper in a non-electronic form, please contact the editorial office:

Editorial Office:	**Editorial Office for submissions from USA and Canada:**
Eva Aralikatti	Tracy Crow
jvr@karger.ch	jvr@tamu.edu
Tel. +49 89 5996 388	Tel. +1 979 458 2782
Fax +49 89 5996 378	Fax +1 979 862 4638

Conditions

All manuscripts are subject to editorial review. Manuscripts are received with the explicit understanding that they are not under simultaneous consideration by any other publication. Submission of an article for publication implies transfer of the copyright from the author to the publisher upon acceptance. Accepted papers become the permanent property of *Journal of Vascular Research* and may not be reproduced by any means, in whole or in part, without the written consent of the publisher. It is the author's responsibility to obtain permission to reproduce illustrations, tables, etc. from other publications.

Sections

Research Papers: Submitted manuscripts should be fully documented reports of original research. They must describe significant and original observations which can be critically evaluated and, if necessary, repeated.

Review: Reviews concerned with topics of current interest in vascular research will be welcome. Potential authors are asked to contact the editors before submitting their papers in order to avoid clashes with other pending reviews. All reviews will be subjected to normal critical peer refereeing.

New Methods in Vascular Research: Primarily methodological papers of interest to the average reader.

Rapid Communication: Manuscripts intended as rapid communications must present new and exciting results of sufficient importance to justify their accelerated acceptance. They should follow the normal arrangement of research papers, including an abstract not exceeding 150 words. Rapid communications should not be more than 3 printed pages in length (including figures, tables and references). Rapid communications can only be accepted as they are or with minor modifications. Rejected manuscripts can only be reconsidered as regular papers. Review will be rapid, and, once accepted, the paper will be included in the next planned issue.

Commentary: Comments concerning current topics of interest in vascular science will be considered for publication by the Editors. They should not be more than one printed page in length (approx. 6,460 characters, spaces included).

Letter to the Editor: Letters to the Editor concerning articles published in *Journal of Vascular Research* may be submitted for publication. If accepted, the authors of the articles concerned will be given the opportunity to reply.

Arrangement

Manuscript organization: Manuscripts should include, in sequence and on separate pages: title and authors, address, running title and acknowledgment of support; abstract and key words; introduction; methods; results; discussion; acknowledgments; references; tables; figures. The normal maximum length is 10 printed pages (including tables, illustrations and references), one printed page containing approximately 6,460 characters, spaces included.

Title page: The first page of each paper should indicate the title, the authors' names, the institute where the work was conducted, and a short title for use as running head.
N.B. Authors wishing to preserve the phonetic meaning of diacritics (PubMed reduces diacritics to their root characters) must spell their names accordingly when submitting manuscripts (e.g. Müller should be Mueller).

Full address: The exact postal address of the corresponding author complete with postal code must be given at the bottom of the title page. Please also supply phone and fax numbers, as well as an e-mail address.

Key words: For indexing purposes, a list of 3–10 key words in English is essential. Consult previous numbers of Journal of Vascular Research for suitable entries.

Abstract: Each paper needs an abstract of up to 200 words.

Footnotes: Acknowledgment of support is printed as a footnote to the title. Other footnotes should be avoided.

Style: All measurements should normally be in SI units. Blood pressure may be given in mm Hg. Use generic names of drugs. Avoid jargon, euphemisms and abbreviations.

Tables and illustrations: Tables and illustrations (both numbered in Arabic numerals) should be prepared on separate pages. Tables require a heading and figures a legend, also prepared on a separate page. Due to technical reasons, figures with a screen background should not be submitted. When possible, group several illustrations in one block for reproduction (max. size 180 × 223 mm) or provide crop marks. Each illustration must be labelled with its number and the first author's name. b/w halftone and color illustrations must have a final resolution of 300 dpi after scaling (final size), line drawings one of 800–1,200 dpi. Figure files must not be embedded in a document file but submitted separately (see detailed instructions at **http://oper.karger.com/jvr/**).

References: In the text identify references by Arabic numerals [in square brackets]. Material submitted for publication but not yet accepted should be noted as 'unpublished data' and not be included in the reference list. The list of references should include only those publications which are cited in the text. Do not alphabetize; number references in the order in which they are first mentioned in the text. The surnames of the authors followed by initials should be given. There should be no punctuation other than a comma to separate the authors. Preferably, please cite all authors. Abbreviate journal names according to the Index Medicus system. (Also see International Committee of Medical Journal Editors: Uniform requirements for manuscripts submitted to biomedical journals. N Engl J Med 1997;336:309–315 or **www.icmje.org**)

Digital Object Identifier (DOI)
S. Karger Publishers supports DOIs as unique identifiers for articles. A DOI number will be printed on the title page of each article. DOIs can be useful in the future for identifying and citing articles published online without volume or issue information. More information can be found at **www.doi.org**

Examples
(a) Papers published in periodicals: Chatel J-M, Bernard H, Orson FM: Isolation and characterization of two complete Ara h 2 isoforms cDNA. Int Arch Allergy Immunol 2003;131:14–18.
(b) Papers published only with DOI numbers: Theoharides TC, Boucher W, Spear K: Serum interleukin-6 reflects disease severity and osteoporosis in mastocytosis patients. Int Arch Allergy Immunol DOI: 10.1159/000063858.
(c) Monographs: Matthews DE, Farewell VT: Using and Understanding Medical Statistics, ed 3, revised. Basel, Karger, 1996.
(d) Edited books: Cochrane AL, Ricardo SD: Oxidant stress and regulation of chemokines in the development of renal interstitial fibrosis; in Razzaque MS, Taguchi T (eds): Renal Fibrosis. Contrib Nephrol. Basel, Karger, 2003, vol 139, pp 102–119.

Video Files

Video files for the Journal of Vascular Research enhance the online versions. The printed journal remains the archival version. Since it does not contain video files, the latter can only be supplements which improve the reader's understanding of the paper. In the printed version they should be replaced by a 'typical' figure. For further information, please refer to **http://oper.karger.com/jvr/**

Color Illustrations

Up to 6 color illustrations per page can be integrated within the text at the special price of CHF 660.–/USD 545.00 per page. Color illustrations are reproduced at the author's expense. Where an author is unable to pay these charges, they may be waived at the discretion of the Editors.

Page Charges

Authors are charged CHF 75.–/USD 53.00 per printed page. 1 printed page is equal to approximately 2 manuscript pages (approx. 6,460 characters, spaces included).

Copy Editing

All manuscripts accepted for publication by Karger are subject to copy editing. Changes introduced by the copy editor and/or questions will be marked in the manuscript so please be sure to check the galleys against the manuscript. The copy edited manuscript will be returned along with the proofs.

Proofs

Unless indicated otherwise, proofs are sent to the first-named author and should be returned with the least possible delay. Alterations made in proofs, other than the correction of printer's errors, are charged to the author. No page proofs are supplied.

Reprints

Order forms and a price list are sent with the proofs. Orders submitted after the issue is printed are subject to considerably higher prices.

KARGER

Fax +41 61 306 12 34
E-Mail karger@karger.ch
www.karger.com

© 2004 S. Karger AG, Basel

The Guidelines for Authors are available at:
www.karger.com/jvr_Guidelines

Journal of Vascular Research

Abstracts

23rd Conference of the European Society for Microcirculation

Microcirculation and Vascular Biology: A Basis for Research and a Reason for Life

Lisbon, Portugal, September 8–11, 2004

Guest Editors
Carlota Saldanha, Lisbon
Axel Pries, Berlin
Victor Oliveira, Lisbon

KARGER
Basel · Freiburg · Paris · London · New York · Bangalore · Bangkok · Singapore · Tokyo · Sydney

S. Karger
Medical and Scientific Publishers
Basel • Freiburg • Paris • London
New York • Bangalore • Bangkok
Singapore • Tokyo • Sydney

Drug Dosage
The authors and the publisher have exerted every effort to ensure that drug selection and dosage set forth in this text are in accord with current recommendations and practice at the time of publication. However, in view of ongoing research, changes in government regulations, and the constant flow of information relating to drug therapy and drug reactions, the reader is urged to check the package insert for each drug for any change in indications and dosage and for added warnings and precautions. This is particularly important when the recommended agent is a new and/or infrequently employed drug.

All rights reserved.
No part of this publication may be translated into other languages, reproduced or utilized in any form or by any means, electronic or mechanical, including photocopying, recording, microcopying, or by any information storage and retrieval system, without permission in writing from the publisher or, in the case of photocopying, direct payment of a specified fee to the Copyright Clearance Center (see 'General Information').

© Copyright 2004 by S. Karger AG,
P.O. Box, CH–4009 Basel (Switzerland)
Printed in Portugal by Colprinter, São João da Talha
ISBN 3–8055–7814–8

KARGER

Fax +41 61 306 12 34
E-Mail karger@karger.ch
www.karger.com

Wednesday, 8 September 2004

Room2	09.00 13.00	**ESM Executive Meeting**
Auditorium	14.00 14.15	**Opening Address** *J. Martins e Silva*, Dean of Lisbon Faculty of Medicine, Portugal *F. Ramoa Ribeiro*, President of the Foundation for Science and Technology, Portugal *C. Saldanha*, President of the European Society for Microcirculation, Portugal *A.R. Pries*, Secretary of the European Society for Microcirculation, Germany *A. Shore*, Treasurer of the European Society for Microcirculation, UK *Braz Nogueira*, Vice-President of the Portuguese Society of Hemorheology and Microcirculation, Portugal *V. Oliveira*, Secretary of the Portuguese Society of Hemorheology and Microcirculation, Portugal & Presentation of the **ESM Travel Awards, International Institute for Microcirculation Award, Travel Award of the German Society for Microcirculation and Vascular Biology**
Auditorium	14.15 15:00	**Plenary Lecture** **Perspectives of Microcirculation** *Giuseppe Ambrosio,* University of Perugia, Italy
Auditorium	15.00 16.45	**Plenary Symposium** **Illusion of Reperfusion: Microvascular Integrity as the Key Factor in Successful Post-ischemic Reperfusion** Chairmen: *Giuseppe Ambrosio*, University of Perugia, Italy *Michael Menger*, Saarland University, Germany Presentations: 1. No-reflow phenomenon: from bench to bedside *Isabella Tritto*, University of Perugia, Italy 2. The origins of the mechanism for leukocyte recruitment/activation in a postischemic microcirculation: application to shock and multiorgan failure *Geert W. Schmid-Schönbein*, University of California, USA 3. Contrast echocardiography to investigate no-reflow patients *Eric Brochet*, Hospital Bichat, France 4. Clinical utility of magnetic resonance imaging *Bernhard L. Gerber*, Cliniques St. Luc UCL, Belgium
	16.45 17.00	Coffee-Break
Auditorium	17.00 18.30	**Plenary Symposium** **Microcirculatory Mechanisms of Hypertension** Chairmen: *Eric Vicaut*, France *Giuseppe Ambrosio*, University of Perugia, Italy 1. Angiogenesis and Hypertension. Basis for a unifying hypothesis? *Harry Struijker Boudier*, Maastricht University, The Netherlands 2. Vascular oxidative stress pro-inflammation in various models of hypertension. Are there common (unifying) mechanisms? *Akos Koller*, Semmelweis University, Hungary 3. Hypothesis derived from the study of microvasculature in patients. *Enrico Agabiti-Rosei*
Hall 01, 1	18.30 20.00	Welcome Reception Porto offered by Lisbon Town Hall

Thursday, 9 September 2004

Auditorium	08.30 09.15	**Plenary Lecture** **Microvascular Mechanisms for Inflammation and Organ Injury in Hypertension** *Geert W. Schmid-Schönbein*, University of California, USA
Auditorium		Presentation of the **JVR/ESM Award, Servier Award in Microcirculation**

Auditorium	09.15 10.45	**Plenary Symposium** **Clinical Microcirculation** Chairman: *Can Ince*, Academic Medical Center, The Netherlands. 1. The microcirculatory response to wound healing following maxillofacial surgery *Jerome Lindeboom*, Academic Medical Center, The Netherlands. 2. Sublingual and intestinal microcirculatory in critically ill patients *Christian Boerma*, Leuwaarden Medical Center, The Netherlands 3. Microcirculation disturbances in heart and lung during open heart surgery *Keshen Mathura*, Academic Medical Center, Amsterdam, The Netherlands 4. The microcirculation during shock and resuscitation *Can Ince*, Academic Medical Center, The Netherlands
	10.45 11.00	Coffee-Break
Auditorium	11.00 12.30	**Plenary Symposium** **Critical Experimental Studies: A More Effective Way to Translate Basic Research Into Therapeutic Options?** *Sponsored by Gesellschaft für Mikrozirkulation und Vaskuläre Biologie E.V.* Chairmen: *Harry Struijker Boudier*, Maastricht University, The Netherlands *Dirk Seiffge*, Aventis Pharma, GmbH, Germany 1.The Problem: Costly failures of clinical studies based on promising experimental data (examples antithrombotic therapy, ischaemia/reperfusion...) *Dirk Seiffge*, Aventis Pharma, GmbH, Germany 2. The Facts: The ischaemia/reperfusion story as an example for failures in development of pharmaceutical strategies *J.M. Harlan*, University of Washington, USA 3. The Analysis: Development of new drugs - structures, mechanisms, and costs in different phases *Harry Struijker Boudier*, Maastricht University, The Netherlands 4. The Approach: Critical experimental studies *Axel R. Pries*, Charité - Universitätsmedizin Berlin, Germany Panel Discussion Final statement *Harry Struijker Boudier*, Maastricht University, The Netherlands
	12.30 13.30	Lunch
Hall 1	13.30 14.15	Guided Poster Tour
Auditorium	14.15 14.45	Introductory Overview Sessions
Auditorium	14.45 16.00	**Free Oral Communications "Assessment Techniques and others"** Chairman: *João Carvalho de Sousa*, Lisbon Faculty of Medicine, Portugal OAT1 *Estimation of O2 Consumption Rate of Arteriolar Walls in Skeletal Muscle* *Masahiro Shibata*, University of Tokyo, Japan OAT2 *A New Model For in vivo Evaluation of Microvascular Reactivity in Man. The Effects of Angiotensin II.* *A.J.H.M. Houben*, University Hospital Maastricht, Maastricht, The Netherlands.

		OAT3 *Two-photon laser scanning microscopic imaging of wall structures in large mouse arteries* *R.T.A Megens*, University of Maastricht, Maastricht, The Netherlands. OAT4 *Using Fibered Confocal Fluorescence Microscopy (Cell-viZioTM) for extended imaging capabilities in the field of microcirculation. Complementarities with intravital microscopy.* *Elisabeth Laemmel*, F. Widal Hospital, Paris, France OAT6 *Are Direct And Indirect Capillary Pressure Measurements Comparable?* *J.C. de Graaff*, St. Antonius Hospital, Nieuwegein; Amsterdam, The Netherlands OAT7 *Simultaneous Monitoring of Oxygenation, Blood Flow, Metabolic Parameters And Nitric Oxide in/From Small Areas of The Rat Brain by Visible Spectroscopy And Laser Doppler* *F.A. Martín*, Fac. de Medicina. Univ. de La Laguna, Tenerife, Islas Canarias, Spain.
	16.00 16.15	Coffee-Break
Room 1	16.15 17.45	**Parallel Symposia** PAS1 : **Retinal Microcirculation: Experimental and Clinical Aspects** Chairmen: *Eric Vicaut*, France *Alon Harris*, Indiana University School of Medicine, USA 1. New insights in structure and function of retinal microvascular networks from in vivo microscopy and 3D reconstruction from confocal images of retina *M. Paques* 2. New techniques for exploration of retinal structure: importance for clinical management of patients *A. Gaudric* Part 2: 1. Vascular risk factors in glaucoma *Luis Metzner Serra*, Lisbon Faculty of Medicine, Portugal 2. Vascular risks in AMD *Alon Harris*, Indiana University School of Medicine, USA 3. Roundtable discussion on clinical significance of vascular risk factors in glaucoma and age related macular degeneration. *Alon Harris*, *Luis Metzner Serra*, *Antonio Castanheira-Dinis*
Room 3	16.15 17.45	PAS2 : **Red Blood Cell Interaction with Blood Vessel Wall Endothelium in Circulatory Disorders** Chairman: *Saul Yedgar*, Jerusalem, Israel 1. Analysis of Hemodynamic Implications of RBC Interactions with Microvascular Endothelium *Alexander Popel*, Baltimore, USA 2. Multifactorial Nature of Sickle Red Cell Adhesion to Vascular Endothelium *Dhanajaya Kaul*, New York, USA 3. Role of ICAM-4 in Red Cell Adhesion to Endothelium *David Anstee*, Bristol, UK 4. Inflammatory mediators promote Red Blood Cell adhesion to endothelium under venular flow conditions *Timothy Wick*, Atlanta, USA 5. RBC Membrane Components in Interaction with Endothelial Cells: Relative Contribution and Interrelation *Saul Yedgar*, Jerusalem, Israel

Auditorium	16.15 17.45	PAS3 : **Microvascular Assessment: Advanced Techniques for Intravital Microscopy** *Sponsored by Gesellschaft für Mikrozirkulation und Vaskuläre Biologie E.V.* Chairmen: *Dick W. Slaaf*, Maastricht University, The Netherlands *Axel R. Pries*, Charité - Universitätsmedizin Berlin, Germany 1. Why intravital microscopy? *Michael Menger*, Saarland University, Germany 2. New techniques: one approach fits all? *Dick W. Slaaf*, Maastricht University, The Netherlands 3. Two-photon microscopy in large and small vessels *Marc van Zandvoort*, Maastricht University, The Netherlands 4. Do they work together? Two-photon microscopy of microvessels and neurons in the brain *Serge Charpak*, ESPCI, Lab. of Neurophysiology, France 5. Seeing is believing: functional tracers *Wolfgang Kübler*, Charité - Universitätsmedizin Berlin, Germany
Room 2	16.15 17.45	PAS4 : **Physiological versus Pathological Angiogenesis: common themes and new perspectives** Chairman: *António J. Cidadão*, Lisbon Faculty of Medicine, Portugal 1. Molecular signaling during normal blood vessel development *Domingos Henrique*, Lisbon Faculty of Medicine, Portugal 2. Molecular basis of endothelial differentiation and tumor angiogenesis *Sérgio Dias*, Gulbenkian Institute of Science, Portugal 3. Physiological *versus* pathological angiogenesis - Round table *António J. Cidadão*, Lisbon Faculty of Medicine, Portugal, *Domingos Henrique*, Lisbon Faculty of Medicine, Portugal, *Sérgio Dias*, Gulbenkian Institute of Science, Portugal
Room 2	17.45 18.15	Meet the Expert
Room 1	18.15	AGM-ESM Business Meeting

Friday, 10 September 2004

Auditorium	08.30 09.15	**Malpighi Award Lecture** **Mechanical and electrical modes of cell-cell interactions in the microcirculation** *Brian Duling*, University of Virginia School of Medicine, USA
Auditorium		Presentation of the **Malpighi Award and Van Leeuwenhoek Awards**
Auditorium	09.15 10.45	**Plenary Symposium** **Gap Junctions and Vascular Cell Communication** Chairmen: *Ulrich Pohl*, Universität München, Germany *Jeremy Pearson*, Centre Vascular Biology & Medicine, UK 1. Gap junctions and endothelium-dependent hyperpolarisation *Tudor Griffith*, Cardiff, UK 2. Nitric oxide and regulation of gap junctions *Ulrich Pohl*, Universität München, Germany 3. Conducted vasodilatation *Cor de Wit*, University of Lubeck, Germany 4. Biochemical characterization of EDHFs *Ingrid Fleming*, Frankfurt, Germany
	10.45 11.00	Coffee-Break

Auditorium	11.00 12.30	**Plenary Symposium** **Programming of Vascular Dysfunction** *Sponsored by British Microcirculation Society* Chairmen: *Christopher Torrens*, University of Southampton, UK *Geraldine F. Clough*, University of Southampton, UK 1. Fetoplacental vascular function in diabetic pregnancy *Jamie Coleman*, University of Dundee, UK 2. Fetal Endothelial Development and Fetal Vascular Control *Eduardo Villamor*, University of Maastricht, Netherlands 3. Programming of Endothelial Dysfunction in utero: Role of Superoxide Anion, Nitric Oxide and Angiotensin II *Maria do Carmo Pinho Franco*, University of São Paulo, Brazil 4. Clinical Implications of Endothelial Dysfunction in low birth weight subjects *Mikael Norman*, Karolinska Institute, Sweden 5. Transgenerational Programming of Endothelial Function *Christopher Torrens*, University of Southampton, UK
	12.30 13.30	Lunch
Hall 01	13.30 14.15	Guided Poster Tour
Auditorium	14.15 14.45	Introductory Overview Sessions
Auditorium	14.45 16.00	**Free Oral Communications Ischemia, Reperfusion** Chairmen: *Dinis da Gama*, Lisbon Faculty of Medicine, Portugal *Victor Oliveira*, Lisbon Faculty of Medicine, Portugal OIR1 Ischemic Preconditioning Improves The Intestinal Oxygenation in Reperfusion Injury of The Intestine, *Ismail H.Mallick*, Royal Free and University College Medical School, United Kingdom OIR2 Platelet-leucocyte and platelet-neutrophil aggregates are markers of the inflammatory response following intermittent claudication, *S Pasupathy*, Vascular Surgical Unit, Leeds General Infirmary, UK OIR3 Inhibition of Rho Kinase Improves Vascular Enos Function During Renal Ischemia Reperfusion, *A.M.G. Versteilen*, Institute for Cardiovascular Research, VU University Medical Center, The Netherlands OIR4 The Effects of Melatonin on Ischemia Reperfusion Injury in Rat Pial Microcirculation, *Antonio Colantuoni*, University Medical School, Italy OIR5 The Effect of Ischaemic Preconditioning on Tissue Oxygenation and Mitochondria Function ofThe Fatty Liver, *Wenxuan Yang*, University Department of Surgery, Royal Free and University College Medical School, United Kingdom OIR6 The endogenous inhibitor of nitric oxide synthase, asymetric dimethilarginine (ADMA) inhibits flow dependent dilation of isolated arterioles, *János Tóth*, Semmelweis University, Hungary OIR7 Vasopressin Treatment in hemorrhagic shock, *Anthony T. Cheung*, University of California, U.S.A.
	16.00 16.15	Coffee-Break

Room 2	16.15 17.45	**Parallel Symposia – PAS** PAS5 : **Cerebral Vascular Disease** Chairmen: *José Ferro*, Lisbon Faculty of Medicine, Portugal *Victor Oliveira*, Lisbon Faculty of Medicine, Portugal Introduction *Victor Oliveira*, Lisbon Faculty of Medicine, Portugal 1. TACIP study *Victor Oliveira*, Lisbon Faculty of Medicine, Portugal 2. Meta-analysis of Triflusal studies *João Costa*, Santa Maria Hospital, Portugal 3. Anti-aggregation and Blood Pressure *Carlos Navas*, Uriach-Barcelona, Spain 4. Triflusal in prevention of cardio-embolism *Francisco Pérez Gómez*, Hospital Clínico San Carlos, Spain Conclusion *José Ferro*, Lisbon Faculty of Medicine, Portugal
Room 1	16.15 17.45	PAS6 : **Leukocyte Trafficking in Inflammation and Disease** *Sponsored by Gesellschaft für Mikrozirkulation und Vaskuläre Biologie E.V.* Chairmen: *Barbara Walzog*, Ludwig-Maximilians-Universität, Germany *Markus Sperandio*, Universitäts-Kinderklinik, Germany 1. Leukocyte trafficking to sites of inflammation: overlapping functions of chemokine receptors and E-selectin *Klaus Ley*, University of Virginia, USA 2. Comparative analysis of T lymphocyte interaction with microvessels in the cerebral cortex and the spinal cord in vivo *Britta Engelhardt*, Theodor-Kocher Institute, Switzerland 3. Inappropriate Leukocyte Activation in Vasculitis and Disseminated Intravascular Coagulation *Keith Norman*, University of Sheffield, UK 4. L-selectin dependent rolling in alpha 2,3-sialyltransferase-IV deficient mice *Markus Sperandio*, Universitäts-Kinderklinik, Germany 5. Involvement of the tyrosine kinase Syk in the control of leukocyte polarization *Jürgen Schymeinsky*, Universität München, Germany
Room 3	16.15 17.45	PAS7 : **Pressure Measurements in Human Microvessels: Fancy or Future?** *Sponsored by Netherlands Society for Microcirculation and Vascular Biology* Chairmen: *J. Tooke*, Peninsula Medical School, UK *D.Th. Ubbink*, University of Amsterdam, The Netherlands 1. Development and principle of the servo-nulling technique in capillary pressure measurements. *D.W. Slaaf*, Cardiovascular Research Institute Maastricht, The Netherlands 2. What information about microcirculatory physiology have we gained from capillary pressure measurements? *C.C. Michel*, Imperial College School of Medicine, UK 3. The clinical significance of capillary blood pressure measurements in the fingers *A.C. Shore*, Exeter University, UK 4. What can we learn from capillary blood pressures in patients with leg ischaemia? *J.C. de Graaff*, Nieuwegein, The Netherlands 5. The relevance of pressure measurements in lymphatic capillaries *B. Amann-Vesti*, Universitätsspital Zürich, Switzerland General Discussion

Room 2	17.45 18.15	Meet the Expert

Saturday, 11 September 2004

Auditorium	08.30 09.00	Introductory Overview Sessions
Auditorium	09.00 10.15	**Free Oral Communications: Angiogenesis Pharmacology and Gene Therapy** Chairman: *José Fernandes e Fernandes*, Lisbon Faculty of Medicine, Portugal OAP1 *Blood Flow Dynamics And Intravascular Oxygen Tension of Tumor Microvessels Under Photodynamic Treatment,* *Haruyuki Minamitani*, Keio University, Yokohama, Japan OAP2 *High Intraluminal Pressure Upregulates Arterial NAD(P)H Oxidase And Renin Angiotensin System Via Protein Kinsase C,* *Akos Koller*, Semmelweis University, Hungary OAP3 *Cardiotonic Pill® improves ischemia-reperfusion-induced microcirculatory disturbances in rat mesentery,* *JingYan Han*, Keio. Universitokyo Tokyo, Japan OAP4 *Intravital investigation of the effects of an anti-vascular and an anti-angiogenic agent on tumour Microvasculature,* *Luciano Andre Guerreiro Lucas*, Cancer Institute, Northwood, UK OAP5 *Effects of an anti-angiogenic agent on growing tumour microvasculature: an intravital investigation,* *Luciano Andre Guerreiro Lucas*, Cancer Institute, Northwood, UK OAP6 *Arterial Collateral Formation Influenced by Cycloidal Vibration,* *P. Lievens*, Vrije University Brussel, Belgium OAP7 *Fibrin is a Potent Stimulus of Endothelial Migration,* *M. Potter*, Mount Vernon Hospital, Northwood London UK
Hall 01	10.15 11.00	Guided Poster Tour
	11.00 11.15	Coffee-Break
Room 2	11.15 12.45	**Parallel Symposia – PAS** PAS8 : **Molecular Mechanisms of Atherosclerosis** *Sponsored by the Portuguese Atherosclerosis Society with an educational grant of Laboratórios Pfizer* Chairmen: *Manuel Carrageta*, Lisbon Faculty of Medicine, Portugal *Jacinto Gonçalves*, Curry Cabral Hospital, Portugal 1. Arterial Hypertension and atherosclerosis: epidemiological aspects *Mário Espiga de Macedo*, Porto Faculty of Medicine, Portugal 2.From endothelial dysfunction to vascular dynamic in risk stratification and therapeutic *Pedro Marques da Silva*, Santa Marta Hospital, Portugal 3. Inflammation and atherosclerosis: the role of reactive C protein *José Manuel Silva*, Coimbra Faculty of Medicine, Portugal 4. Recommendations to change the clinical practice *Armando Serra Coelho*, Instituto Cardiologia Preventiva, Portugal

Room 1	11.15 12.45	PAS9 : **Molecular Imaging of Apoptosis in the Vessel Wall** *Sponsored by Netherlands Society for Microcirculation and Vascular Biology* Chairmen: *Leo Hofstra*, University Hospital Maastricht, the Netherlands *A. Houben*, Cardiovascular Research Institute Maastricht, the Netherlands 1. Annexin-V and molecular imaging: how to develop a probe for imaging cell death *C. Reutelingsperger*, University of Maastricht, The Netherlands 2. Molecular imaging of the unstable plaque *J. Narula*, Irvine Medical Center, USA 3. Imaging of apoptosis in patients with cardiovascular disease *L. Hofstra*, University Hospital Maastricht, the Netherlands 4. Microvascular apoptosis *A. Houben*, Cardiovascular Research Institute Maastricht, the Netherlands
Auditorium	11.15 12.45	PAS10 : **Frontiers in Angiogenesis: Mechanisms and Applications** Chairmen: *G. Molema*, Groningen, The Netherlands *Michael Weis*, Klinikum Großhadern, German 1. The role of hemodynamics and neuronal guidance molecules in arterial-venous differentiation and patterning *Ferdinand le Noble*, Maastricht University, The Netherlands 2. Stem cells and progenitor cells in postnatal neovascularization: Molecular mechanisms and clinical relevance *Christopher Heeschen*, University Clinic, Germany 3. Antiangiogenic therapies and targeted strategies *G. Molema*, Groningen, The Netherlands 4. Therapeutic angiogenesis: quo vadis? *Christian Kupatt*, Klinikum Großhadern, Germany
Room 3	11.15 12.45	PAS11 : **From Endothelial Dysfunction to Atherothrombosis** Chairmen: *José Fernandes e Fernandes*, Lisbon Faculty of Medicine, Portugal *Luis Mendes Pedro*, Lisbon Faculty of Medicine, Portugal 1. Flow mediated vasodilatation and the shear stress paradox: Is exercise harmful? *William Paaske*, Denmark 2. NO as a marker of endothelial dysfunction: clinical Correlations *Carlota Saldanha*, Lisbon Faculty of Medicine, Portugal 3. Oxidative Stress and Inflammation modulate vascular function in Hypermocysteinemia (HHCY) *Akos Koller*, Semmelweis University, Hungary 4. "In vivo" identification of the "vulnerable" atheromatous plague *Luis Mendes Pedro*, Lisbon Faculty of Medicine, Portugal 5. Overview: Clinical implications and treatment options *José Fernandes e Fernandes*, Lisbon Faculty of Medicine, Portugal
Auditorium	12.45 13.30	Invitation to next ESM Meeting Amsterdam 2006

Grady, M.	PAT.2
Grieb, P.	PIR.1
Griffioen, A.W.	PAN.3
Groeneveld, A.B.J	OIR.3
Guerra, J.	POP.10
Gunther, R.A,	OIR.7
Guven, S.F.	POP.6
Haigh, R.C.	PEF.11
Hajizadeh, S.	PHD.7
Hampton, S.M.	PEF.8,PEF.9
Han, JingYan	OAP.3
Hannemann, M.M.	PEF.12
Harper, S. J.	PAN.4
Hartmann, K.	POS.3, POS.4
Haskard, D.O.	PEB.2
Hawary, Sherif El	PDM.4
Hewinson, James	PIN.6
Hibi, T.	OAP.3
Hill, S.A.	OAP.4, PTV.2
Hinz, B.	PAT.3
Hollenberg M.D.	PIN.4
Homentcovschi C.	PHT.1
Honess, D.	PTV.2
Horrocks, M.	PIN.6
Hoseong Lee	PHT.2
Houben, A.J.H.M.	OAT.2
Huang, Miao-Tzu	PEB.2
Ichioka, S.	OAT.1
Ileri, E.	POP.6
Ireson, Christopher R.	PTV.2
Isaksson, B.	PAN.1
Ishii, H.	OAP.3
Itoh, Y.	PBC.1
Iwata, Y.	OAP.1
Jahr, J.S.	OIR.7
James, L.	PEF.8
Jankovec Z.	PDM.6
Járai, Z.	PEF.6
Jiang, K.	OAP.4,OAP.5
Jiang, Xucheng	PSM.1
Kajiya, F.	POP.4
Kaley, G	PDM.7
Kamiya A .	OAT.1
Kanthou, C.	PTV.2
Karagiannis, E.D.	PAN.2
Kasalová, Z.	PAD.1
Kelso, E.B.	PEF.1, PIN.4
Kikuchi, H. E.	PIN.8
Kikuchi, Yuji	PIN.8
Kiss, I .	PEF.6
Koeppen, K.B.M.	PEF.10
Kohzuki, H.	POP.4
Koller, Akos	PDM.7, OAP.2, OIR.6
Kolossváry, E.	PEF.6
Kono Ichiro	PHT.2
Konopatskaya, Olga	PAN.4
Koopman B.	PAD.3
Korstjens, I.	OIR.3

Kraus, J.	PEB.3,POS.3,POS.4
Krcma, M.	PDM.6
Kristóf, V.	PTO.1
Kroner,C.	PHD.1
Kronschnabl, M.	PEF.14
Kulawik, T.	PIR.1
Kurosu, T.	PIN.8
Kwee, L.	PAN.3
Kylander, C.	PAN.1
Lacigova, S.	PDM.6
Laczkó, Á.	PTO.1
Laemmel Elisabeth	OAT.4, POS.1
Lambrecht, S.	POF.1
Lapi, D.	OIR.4
Leach, L.	PEB.4
Lee, B.	PEF.12
Leeuw P.W. de	OAT.2
Legemate, D.A .	PAD.2
Lehr H.A.	PIN.2
Lewis, G.	PTV.2
LI, Wenjun	PSM.1
Liao, James K.	PEB.1
Liddell, W.	PEF.12
Lidington, E.	PEB.2
Liedl, D.A.	POP.5
Lievens, P.	OAP.6
Lindberg, L-G.	PHD.10
Linge, C.	OAP.7, PEB.6
Lockhart J.C.	PAT.2, PEF.1, PIN.3, PIN.4, PIN.5
Lourenço, M.	PHT.3
Lucas, Luciano Andre Guerreiro	OAP.4,OAP.5
Luis-García, Mª.L.	PAT.4, PAT.5, OAT.7
Mac Gabhann, F.	PAN.7
MacLoed, K.M.	PDM.8
Mallick I.H.	OIR.1
Marchiafava, P.L.	OIR.4
Maria, A. V.	POP.8, POP.10
Martín, F.A.	PAT.4, PAT.5, OAT.7
Martins e Silva, J.	PAT.6,PBC.2,PBC.3, PBC.4,PEF.15, POP.7, POP.8,POP.9,POP.10, PIN.10, PVF.2
Martins Prata, M.	POP.10
Maskell, L.	PAN.5
Mason, J.C.	PEB.2
Matharan S. Therade	POS.1
Mather, S.	PEF.5
Matsuo, Masato	POP.2
McHarg, S.	PEB.7
Mchedlishvili G.	PCV.1, PHD.4
McLean J.S.	PIN.5
Meawad Rania	PDM.5
Megens, R.T. A .	OAT.3
Melik, Ziva	PHD.5
Merino, C.	OAT.7, PAT.4, PAT.5
Middlebrooke, A.R.	PEF.12

Poster Categories and Codes

Code	Category	Presentation Day
PAD	Microcirculation alterations in atherosclerosis and dyslipidemias	Thursday, 9 Sept
PAN	Angiogenesis and stem cells	Thursday, 9 Sept
PAT	Assessment techniques	Thursday, 9 Sept
PBC	Cell/Vessel Wall Interactions	Thursday, 9 Sept
PCM	Coronary microcirculation	Thursday, 9 Sept
PCV	Microcirculation and cerebral vascular disease	Thursday, 9 Sept
PDM	Microcirculation alterations in diabetes	Thursday, 9 Sept
PEB	Endothelial Cell Biology	Friday, 10 Sept
PEF	Endothelial function and vascular control	Friday, 10 Sept
PHD	Haemodynamics and vascular responses	Friday, 10 Sept
PHT	Haemostasis/thrombosis and platelet function	Friday, 10 Sept
PHY	Hypertension and end-organ damage	Saturday, 11 Sept
PIN	Inflammation/leukocyte function	Saturday, 11 Sept
PIR	Ischemia and reperfusion injury	Saturday, 11 Sept
POF	Microcirculation and ophthalmology	Saturday, 11 Sept
POP	Other pathologies	Saturday, 11 Sept
POS	Oxygen and oxidative stress	Saturday, 11 Sept
PSM	Smooth muscle cell biology	Saturday, 11 Sept
PTO	Treatment options: pharmacology, gene therapy	Saturday, 11 Sept
PTV	Tumor vasculature / biology	Saturday, 11 Sept
PVF	Venous function	Saturday, 11 Sept

PAD 1

MICROVASCULAR REACTIVITY AFTER STATIN TREATMENT IN HYPERLIPIDEMIC DIABETIC AND NON-DIABETIC PATIENTS

M. Prázný, Z. Kasalová, T. Štulc, M. Vrablík, J. Škrha
3rd Department of Internal Medicine, 1st Faculty of Medicine, Charles Univesity, U nemocnice 1, 12808 Prague, Czech Republic

Aims: The aim of the study was to compare the forearm skin microvascular reactivity in Type 2 diabetic patients and non-diabetic subjects with hyperlipidemia before and after statin treatment.

Subjects and methods: 17 Type 2 diabetic patients (D) were treated with 20 mg of simvastatin daily, 21 non-diabetic subjects without proven atherosclerosis (A-) were treated with 20 mg of atorvastatin daily. Skin microvascular reactivity (MVR) following ischemic (PORH) and thermal (TH) stimuli was examined by laser--doppler flowmetry before and after 3 months of treatment. Control group (C) consisted of 20 healthy persons without hyperlipidemia. Maximal perfusion ($PORH_{max}$, TH_{max}) and velocity of perfusion increase ($PORH_{max/t}$, $TH_{max/t}$) were recorded. Study was approved by ethical comittee and consent was obtained from each subject. Paired t-test and ANOVA were used for statistical analysis.

Results. $^{x}p<0.03$ - D group before and after treatment. Data are mean±SD.

	$PORH_{max}$ (PU)		$PORH_{max/t}$ (PU/s)		TH_{max} (PU)		$TH_{max/t}$ (PU/s)	
D	56±30	26±12^{x}	7.7±7.4	2.0±1.4^{x}	135±71	67±19^{x}	1.5±0.7	1.0±0.6^{x}
A-	62±39	62±28	5.2±3.6	4.9±2.2	143±76	147±66	2.1±1.3	2.4±1.1
C	52±20	-	4.0±2.3	-	115±41	-	1.5±0.7	-

Conclusion: There were no statistically significant differences in MVR between the study groups before treatment. After 3 months of statin therapy, a significant decrease in MVR in D group was found. However, there was virtually no change in MVR in A- group despite the profound lipid lowering. The effect of statin treatment on MVR is therefore probably different in diabetic and non-diabetic subjects with hyperlipidemia.

Supported by research project J13/98:111100002.

PAD 2

RANDOMISED STUDY OF THE EFFECT OF GM-CSF ON MACRO- AND MICROCIRCULATION IN INTERMITTENT CLAUDICATION

D.Th. Ubbink[1], B. Atasever[2], N. van Royen[2], D.A. Legemate[1].
Depts. of Vascular Surgery[1] and Cadiology[2], Academic Medical Centre, P.O. Box 22700, 1100 DE, Amsterdam, The Netherlands.

Granulocyte macrophage colony stimulating factor (GM-CSF) is an arteriogenetic agent known to improve collateral blood flow in animal models and patients with coronary artery disease. We investigated whether GM-CSF is also capable of influencing the macro and microcirculation in patients with intermittent claudication (IC).

Patients with invalidating IC (Rutherford grade I, category 2 or 3) were randomised after informed consent. They received either 10 µg/kg GM-CSF or placebo subcutaneously, every other day, for 14 days. Measurements of the ankle blood pressure (AP), ankle/brachial index (ABI), a treadmill test, and laser Doppler perfusion (Periflux PF4001) of the big toes (at rest [LDRF] and during postocclusive hyperaemia[LDPF]) were performed before, and 14 and 90 days after treatment.

Thirty patients, with a mean age of 63 years and of which 20 males, were studied. Both the GM-CF and the placebo group showed a significant increase in walking distance (placebo: from 126±66m tot 189±66m; GM-CSF: from 121±68m to 187±91m). No statistical differences were found between the groups. ABI was not different after treatment in either group. The laser Doppler showed a significant (p=0.02) decrease in time of the hyperaemic perfusion (LDPF minus LDRF) in the placebo group, but not in the GM-CSF treated group.

GM-CSF, as administered in this study, does not improve the clinical, macro-circulatory situation of patients with IC, but does appear to prevent a reduction in microcirculatory flow reserve.

PAD 3

IS NEAR-INFRARED SPECTROSCOPY USEFUL IN THE ROUTINE DIAGNOSTIC WORKUP OF PATIENTS WITH LEG ISCHAEMIA?

D. Th. Ubbink, B. Koopman.
Department of Surgery, Academic Medical Center, P.O. Box 22700, 1100DE, Amsterdam, The Netherlands.

Near infrared spectroscopy (NIRS) is a non-invasive technique to assess tissue oxygen saturation (TsO_2), which could be a valuable additional clinical tool to assess peripheral vascular disease (PVD).

Routinely measured parameters (ankle/brachial index [ABI], toe blood pressure [TBP] and transcutaneous oxygen pressure [TsO_2]) were compared with tissue oxygen saturation (TsO_2) measurements, using a new NIRS device (Inspectra, Hutchinson), and laser Doppler skin perfusion measurements (LDF). These measurements were performed on the calf muscle and on the foot of healthy subjects (n=20) and patients in different stages of PAOD (n=45), at rest and after provocation tests: a treadmill test, arterial occlusion and a change in posture. To assess reproducibility, all measurements were performed twice within 2 weeks in healthy volunteeers.

Calf TsO_2 values were significantly higher in healthy males than females (83% vs. 53%; p<0.001). After exercise, TsO_2 decreased slightly but significantly (p<0.001) to 77% and 48%, respectively). Reproducibility of the NIRS at rest and after exercise was excellent (ICCs of 0.91 and 0.90), as opposed to many other parameters. The PVD patients (mean age 60 years; 19 males, 26 females) were classified according to their Fontaine stage (F). In F1 subjects the resting TsO_2 (65%) did not differ significantly with that in patients (F2 = 66%; F3/4 = 68%). After exercise, a significant reduction in TsO_2 was seen only in PVD patients: F1 = 60% vs. F2 = 21% and F3/4 = 29%. The ABI after exercise showed a good correlation (R=0.73) with TsO_2 at the end of the treadmill test. No correlation between NIRS and other micro- and macrocirculatory parameters was found.

NIRS is a very reproducible tool to assess tissue oxygen saturation. NIRS is able to determine the presence of PVD during exercise, but no relationship with other diagnostic parameters exists. Hence, NIRS does not appear to be a useful additive tool for the routine investigation of patients with leg ischaemia, but adds to our pathophysiological understanding.

PAD 4

RELATION BETWEEN PERIPHERAL PRESSURE MEASUREMENTS AND QUALITY OF LIFE

J.C. de Graaff[1], D.Th. Ubbink[2]
Dept. of Anaesthesiology[1], St. Antonius Hospital, PO Box 2500, 3430EM Nieuwegein; Dept. of Vascular Surgery[2], Academic Medical Center, Amsterdam, The Netherlands.

Transcutaneous oxygen pressure ($TcpO_2$), toe-pressure (TP), ankle pressure (AP) and ankle brachial index (ABI) are frequently measured in the assessment of the severity of peripheral arterial occlusive disease. These variables are also used for the indication for vascular intervention by the vascular surgeon. We investigated before intervention the relation between peripheral pressure measurements and quality of life in 64 patients with critical leg ischaemia (Fontaine stage 3 and 4) requiring vascular intervention.

The correlation between $TcpO_2$, TP, AP, ABI and quality of life (9 domains of SF 36 and the physical and mental summary subscore) and severity of pain (visual analogue scale) was assessed using the Spearman correlation coefficient (rho).

$TcpO_2$ and TP were not related to any of the 11 subscores of quality of life and pain. The AP was only related to physical functioning (rho=0.35, p=0.005), social functioning (rho=0.27, p=0.04). The ABI was only related to physical functioning (rho=0.34, p=0.008), social functioning (rho=0.25, p=0.05).

Peripheral pressure measurements (microvasular and macrovasuclar) are only slightly related to clinical symptoms(quality of life and pain) as experienced by the patient. Only the macrovascular parameters are somewhat related to some aspects of quality of life. Therefore the indication for vascular intervention should be based on the combination of the anamneses of the clinical symptoms (severity of symptoms as experienced by the patient), physical examination, micro, and microvascular peripheral pressure measurements, and duplex and/or angiographic findings.

PAN 1

PATIENTS WITH UNRESECTABLE PANCREATIC CANCER RESPONSE TO IM862.

L. Perbeck, J. Permert, B. Isaksson, C. Kylander.
Department of Surgery, M52, Huddinge University Hospital, 141 86 Stockholm, Sweden.

IM862, manufactured by Cytran Inc, is a bipeptide with antiangiogenetic effects and only minor side effects. The drug is administered as nose drops. The aim of this pilot study was to evaluate the local response of IM862 in patients with locally advanced pancreatic cancer.
Ten patients with unresectable pancreatic cancer with an estimated survival of at least 4 months were included. The patients were examined before and every 3 month by CT-scan and MRI and every month by antigene CA 19-9. IM862 5 mg was taken as nose drops 3 times a day.
Two patients died before they received the treatment. 4 patients died within 4 months. One patient died after 9 months and 3 survived 12 months treatment. If the results are analyzed in the 4 patients who survived 4 months, one showed an initial progression for 3 months wherafter the patient combined the treatment with chemotherapy (Gemsar®), whereafter the tumor showed a stable disease for 9 months according to CT and CA 19-9 values. One patient showed in initial tumor progression for 3 months whereafter there was a stable disease for 9 months. One patient showed a stable disease for 6 months according to CT and CA 19-9 values whereafter there was a progression. In the patient who died after 9 months there was a progression of the tumor all the time including the development of pulmonary metastasis. There were no side effects of the treatment.
IM862 as a single therapy is not enough to prevent progression of pancreatic cancer. There was a period of stable disease for 6-9 months. In the future a combination of antiangiogenetic therapy and chemotherapy might be beneficial.

PAN 2

THE MIGRATING ENDOTHELIAL "TIP" CELL REGULATES DISTINCT PROTEASE ACTIVITIES DURING SPROUTING ANGIOGENESIS: INSIGHTS FROM A THEORETICAL MODEL

A.S. Popel and E.D. Karagiannis
Department of Biomedical Engineering, Johns Hopkins University School of Medicine, Baltimore, 21205 MD, USA.

During angiogenesis, extracellular matrix (ECM) macromolecules are an essential substrate for endothelial cell (EC) migration required for branching morphogenesis. At high density they also pose a physical resistance to the EC movement. Thus the balance between degraded and undegraded matrix is critical for EC migration and subsequent vessel formation.

One important family of enzymes responsible for the ECM degradation are the free diffusing and membrane bound matrix metalloproteinases (MMPs). Recently it has been proposed that during sprouting angiogenesis this proteolytic load is mostly carried out by a single "leading" or "tip" cell, which expresses MMPs to proteolyse the extracellular matrix.

Here we present a computational approach for studying proteolysis of a type I collagen matrix by a moving cell expressing the free diffusing MMP2 and the cell surface localized MT1-MMP in the presence of their inhibitor TIMP2. By virtually "knocking out" the collagenolytic ability of each of the studied enzymes, we provide evidence that matrix proteolysis is localized at the surface of the moving cell and is carried out mostly by MT1-MMPs. This membrane bound MMP-induced proteolysis is sufficient to satisfy the collagenolytic load that will allow the cells to move through the matrix under naturally occurring velocities (2-8 μm/h). The free diffusing MMP2 is not potent enough to support such proteolysis, thus suggesting, for this particular enzyme, alternate roles such as growth factor release from the ECM.

PAN 3

ANTI-ANGIOGENESIS THERAPY CAN OVERCOME ENDOTHELIAL CELL ANERGY AND PROMOTE LEUKOCYTE-VESSEL WALL INTERACTIONS AND INFILTRATION IN TUMORS

A.E.M. Dirkx, M.G.A. oude Egbrink, K. CastermansV.L.J.L. Thijssen, D.W.J. van der Schaft, L. Kwee, J.C.A. Bouma and A.W. Griffioen
Research Intstitutes GROW and CARIM, Maastricht University, P.O. Box 616, 6200 MD Maastricht, the Netherlands

Tumor escape from immunity, as well as the failure of several anti-cancer vaccination and cellular immunotherapy approaches, is suggested to be due to the angiongenesis mediated suppression of endothelial cell (EC) adhesion molecules involved in leukocyte-vessel wall interactions. In the present study we investigated whether inhibition of angiogenesis could overcome this escape from immunity.

Intravital microscopy was used to visualize ear skin microvessels of anesthetized C57Bl/6 mice bearing murine B16F10 melanomas. Leukocyte-vessel wall interactions were quantified both within and outside small tumors growing in the ear. We found that the angiogenesis inhibitors anginex, endostatin and angiostatin, and also the chemotherapeutic agent paclitaxel significantly stimulate leukocyte-vessel wall interactions *in vivo* by circumvention of EC anergy, i.e. by upregulation of endothelial adhesion molecules in tumor vessels. This was confirmed by *in vitro* studies on cultured EC at the protein and mRNA levels. The new angiostatic desgner peptide anginex was most potent at overcoming EC anergy; for this peptide it was shown that the enhanced leukocyte-vessel wall interactions led to an increase in the numbers of tumor infiltrating leukocytes. While anginex inhibited tumor growth and microvessel density significantly, the amount of infiltrated leukocytes (CD45), as well as the number of $CD8^+$ cytotoxic T-lymphocytes, was enhanced markedly.

The current results suggest that anti-cancer immunotherapy strategies can be improved by combination with anti-angiogenesis.

PAN 4

A FAMILY OF INHIBITORY SPLICE VARIANTS OF VEGF ARE EXPRESSED AS PROTEINS IN HUMAN OCULAR TISSUES AND ISOLATED HUMAN RETINAL PIGMENTED EPITHELIAL CELLS

O. Konopatskaya[1], S. J.Harper[1], D.O.Bates[1], A.Churchill[2]
[1]Microvascular Research Laboratories, Department of Physiology, and [2]Bristol Eye Hospital, University of Bristol, Bristol, BS28EJ, UK.

Vascular Endothelial Growth Factor (VEGF) controls pathological angiogenesis and increased vascular permeability in diabetic retinopathy and age-related macular degeneration, and is up-regulated by glucose in retinal cells (Sone et al., BBRC.1996; 221:193-8). The inhibitory splice variant $VEGF_{165}b$ is down-regulated in angiogenic tumours (Bates et al., Cancer Research 2002;62:4123-31) and is anti-angiogenic *in vivo*. We set out to determine whether $VEGF_{165}b$ is expressed in human ocular tissues and retinal pigment epithelial (RPE) cells. Human eyes were obtained within 10-30 hours post-mortem from donors and ocular tissues dissected. RPE was isolated and characterised by immunohisto-chemistry with an anti-cytokeratin antibody. Expression of $VEGF_{165}b$ was revealed in the lysate of RPE cells, retina, iris, lens, sclera and vitreous (n=2-4) by Western blotting with a C-terminal specific anti-body. Multiple bands were detected. These were confirmed to be VEGF isoforms by Western blotting with a commercial pan VEGF antibody. This suggests that multiple $VEGF_{xxx}b$ isoforms were present, eg $VEGF_{121}$ $VEGF_{189}$, $VEGF_{148}$ and large VEGF. Secreted $VEGF_{xxx}b$ in RPE conditioned medium could also be detected by sandwich ELISA (n=4). Furthermore, RT-PCR of RPE RNA using primers flanking the 3'UTR and exon 7 of the mRNA, showed $VEGF_{xxx}b$ mRNA expression. The expression spectrum of VEGF isoforms in human ocular tissues therefore is characterised by the presence of multiple inhibitory splice variants, and potentially may play a significant role in the development of angiogenic eye diseases. Funded by Diabetes UK.

PAN 5

BIO-REDUCTIVE PRODRUG INHIBITION OF VEGF-STIMULATED ANGIOGENESIS

L.Maskell[*], E.Blanche[#], C.J.Moody[#], J.L.Whatmore[*]
[*]Institute for Biomedical and Clinical Sciences, Peninsula Medical School, Exeter, UK. [#] School of Chemistry, University of Exeter, Exeter, UK.

Angiogenesis is essential for tumour growth and metastasis formation and is critically regulated by vascular endothelial growth factor (VEGF). Inhibition of VEGF-induced angiogenesis is a potential anti-tumour therapy. Endothelial cells in tumours over-express reducing enzymes such as NQ01 and cytochrome P450 reductase and it may be possible to exploit these enzymes to target delivery of anti-angiogenic drugs.

Aim: To evaluate the inhibitory potential of "bio-reductive prodrugs" that will release the active anti-angiogenic drug following enzymatic reduction.

Methods: Three delivery systems were designed: 4-nitrobenzyl, 4-nitrobenzyloxycarbonyl and 2-nitrobenzylcarbonyl; and attached to the known anti-angiogenic drugs SU5416 and biochanin A. Prodrugs i.e. drug plus delivery system were tested *in vitro* to examine their inhibition of VEGF-stimulated capillary-like tubule formation. Human umbilical vein endothelial cells were seeded onto fibrin matrices. After 24hrs, drugs or prodrugs (in DMSO) ±VEGF (100ng/ml) were added. Controls received DMSO ±VEGF. Formation of tubular structures was quantified after 48hrs.

Results: SU5416 and biochanin A inhibited angiogenesis by 99.46% at 10μM (p=<0.001, n=15) and 92% at 100μM (p=<0.001, n=9), respectively. The 2-nitrobenzylcarbonyl appears to be a promising delivery system. When bound to SU5416 47% inhibition was observed at 10μM (p=<0.005, n=9) and 100% inhibition was observed when bound to biochanin A at 100μM (p=<0.005, n=9).

Conclusion: Prodrugs of SU5416 and biochanin A and the delivery system 2- nitrobenzylcarbonyl significantly inhibited VEGF-stimulated tubule formation.

PAN 6

HUMAN NEUTROPHILS PROMOTE ANGIOGENESIS: A ROLE FOR HYPOXIA-INDUCILBE FACTOR 1 (HIF-1α)

R. Schruefer and B. Walzog
Dept. of Physiology, Ludwig-Maximilians-Universität, 80336 Munich, Germany.

Human polymorphonuclear neutrophils (PMN) play an important role in host defence and inflammation. The present study was undertaken to investigate the ability of human PMN to promote angiogenesis during the inflammatory response. Using an in vitro angiogenesis assay, we found that activated PMN induced the sprouting of capillary-like structures. To gain further insight into the molecular mechanism underlying this effect, we employed the oligonucleotide microarray technique to identify angiogenesis-relevant genes in human PMN. We detected the expression of > 26 angiogenesis-relevant genes including hypoxia-inducible factor 1 alpha (HIF-1α) in human PMN. This result was confirmed by reverse transcription and polymerase chain reaction (RT-PCR). By means of western blotting technique, HIF-1α was not detectable at the protein level in freshly isolated PMN but it was found to be markedly up-regulated upon culture of human PMN for 6 h and 20 h under hypoxic conditions. Subsequently, we studied the mRNA expres-sion of the HIF-1α-dependent gene vascular endothelial growth factor (VEGF) by RT-PCR and found a substantial up-regulation of the VEGF mRNA upon hypoxia. To study the biological relevance of the observed effect, we used an in vivo angiogenesis assays and found that the conditioned media obtained from human PMN cultured under hypoxic conditions for 6 h or 20 h substantially induced angiogenesis. Taken together, our findings suggest that the inflammatory microenvironment characterised by low-oxygen tension promotes the pro-angiogenic activity of human PMN via up-regulation of HIF-1 α and VEGF. (Supported by DFG WA 1048/1-1)

PAN 7

VASCULAR ENDOTHELIAL GROWTH FACTOR AND VEGF-RECEPTOR FAMILIES: COMPUTATIONAL MODELS OF INTERACTIONS DURING ANGIOGENESIS

A.S. Popel, F. Mac Gabhann
Department of Biomedical Engineering, Johns Hopkins University School of Medicine, 720 Rutland Ave, Baltimore, MD 21205 USA.

The vascular endothelial growth factor (VEGF) family comprises secreted, dimeric glycoproteins that act primarily on endothelial cells and are major mediators of angiogenesis. Multiple receptors for the VEGF family exist on endothelial cells, some of which are VEGF isoform-specific, e.g. Neuropilin-1, which does not initiate signals directly but modulates VEGF binding to signaling VEGF receptors.

We construct computational models of these complex interactions to mimic in vitro and in vivo situations. We validate the models using existing experimental data, and we can reproduce observed in vitro receptor binding and intracellular phosphorylation data. Using the parameters calculated from in vitro models, we predict the in vivo transport of VEGF isoforms. The growth factors are secreted by parenchymal cells and diffuse through the extracellular matrix (to which certain VEGF isoforms bind) to their endothelial cell surface receptors.

Extracellular matrix binding sites are shown not to affect the receptor binding profile in quiescent tissue, and over small distances, not significantly in activated tissue with upregulated VEGF secretion. We examine the relationship between the predicted transport, the establishment of VEGF gradients, and the experimentally observed microvascular changes in tissues expressing specific VEGF isoforms. We also characterize the synergy observed between placental growth factor and VEGF in vitro, and investigate the effect of such synergy in vivo.

These are the first such molecular-level computational models of the VEGF family and their receptors.

PAT 1

COLD SALINE ELICITS PROFOUND AND NON-AUTONOMIC MEDIATED BRADYCARDIA AND HYPOTENSION IN RABBITS

C. I. Wright, E. Thakore, D. Roach, H. Duff, R. S. Sheldon
Cardiovascular Research Group, University of Calgary, Alberta, Canada

Empirically, we observed profound, transient bradycardia's and hypotension to cold saline (CS), but not warm injections in chronic, autonomically intact rabbits. Little is known about such responses and to us they may be useful for assessing the functionality of the autonomic nervous system or even the heart itself. To determine these possibilities, we assessed the effects of selective autonomic blockers on CS mediated responses. In non-sedated New Zealand rabbits, the left central ear artery was canulated and arterial blood pressure (MAP) recorded, the right and left lateral ear veins served as CS injection and drug infusion sites respectively, and an ecg monitored R-R interval (RRi). Peak responses to CS (0-4°C) injections (0.5, 1, 2 and 3ml) were determined before and after muscarinic [0.1mg kg^{-1} of glycopyrrolate(G)], alpha-1 [0.5mg kg^{-1} of prazosin(P)] or beta-receptor blockade [0.5mg kg^{-1} of metoprolol(M)]. CS injections linearly increased RRi and decreased MAP. Prior to G (n=7), CS maximally increased RRi by 224±54ms ($P<0.01$, ANOVA; from 281±6) and decreased MAP by 12.1±2.3mmHg ($P<0.01$; from 67.4±2.1). After G, which decreased resting RRi (-40±5ms; $P<0.05$, paired t test) but not MAP ($P>0.05$), maximal changes in RRi (+117±15ms) and MAP (-6.9±1.0mmHg) were significantly reduced, compared to control ($P<0.05$), but not abolished ($P<0.05$, ANOVA). P (n=4), decreased ($P<0.05$) resting RRi (-29±6ms from 263±10) and MAP (-11.6±2.6mmHg from 69.4±3.9), and maximal responses were not changed ($P<0.05$). M (n=4), increased resting RRi ($P<0.05$; +5±2ms, from 272±7) but resting MAP was unchanged, and maximal RRi and MAP responses were unaffected. To conclude, CS mediates profound bradycardia, which seems to be induced by the heart itself and hence may be useful for testing cardiac function.

PAT 2

IMPROVED SPATIAL RESOLUTION USING NEAR INFRA-RED LASER DOPPLER IMAGING

L. Dunning[1], J.C. Lockhart[1], R. Campbell[1], M. Grady[2], W.R. Ferrell[3]
[1]Biological Sciences, University of Paisley, Paisley PA1 2BE; [2]Inverness Medical Ltd, Beechwood Business Park North, Inverness IV2 3ED; [3]Centre for Rheumatic Diseases, Royal Infirmary, Glasgow G31 2ER; Scotland, UK.

Laser Doppler imaging (LDI) is a relatively recent development permitting two-dimensional mapping of tissue perfusion, imparting greater spatial resolution at the expense of temporal resolution. Standard LDI instruments are equipped with a red laser, but it is known that longer wavelengths have greater penetrating power [Anderson RR & Parrish MD. J Invest Dermatol 1981; 77: 13-17], potentially yielding improved spatial resolution. In this study we compared perfusion at two sites of the upper limb using a laser Doppler imager (Moor Instruments Ltd, Axminster, UK), scanning at red (635nm) and near infra-red (NIR; 835nm) wavelengths simultaneously. The perfusion pattern with either laser was similarly heterogeneous, being greatest at the fingertips and lower over the dorsum of the hand and arm. However, the NIR signal was consistently greater at the fingertips. Most noticeable was the improved definition of the venous pattern using the NIR laser, implying enhanced transcutaneous perfusion imaging. This supports our previous work in which we observed elevated perfusion associated with the inflamed interphalangeal joints of patients with active rheumatoid arthritis [Ferrell WR et al. Radiology, 2001; 220: 257-262]. At both red and NIR wavelengths the signal derived from the fingertip was stable, there being no significant between-day variation ($P = 0.34$ and 0.68 respectively) when measured in three subjects on three separate days. Whilst LDI yields stable measurements, care must be exercised with patient recruitment in studies examining peripheral perfusion. An extreme example that illustrates this is the menopausal 'hot flush', as observed in one subject in whom perfusion was found to increase by over 100%.

PAT 3

MEASUREMENT OF OXYGEN SATURATION IN MESENTERIC MICROVESSELS DURING INTRAVITAL MICROSCOPY USING A MULTISPECTRAL IMAGING SYSTEM.

B. Styp-Rekowska, A.J.M. Cornelissen, B. Reglin, N. Mecha Disassa, B. Hinz, A.R. Pries
Dept. of Physiology, Charité CBF, Berlin, Germany

Introduction: Structural and functional characteristics of microvascular networks are continuously adapting to changing metabolic and hemodynamic conditions. This process has been called angioadaptation. In angiogenesis and angioadaptation the local availability of oxygen plays a pivotal role. Thus, angiogenesis research is one area where the assessment of oxygen saturation (SO_2) in microvessels during intravital microscopy, is of interest. Methods: An intravital microscope connected to an imaging system (T.I.L.L. Photonics, Gräfelfing, Germany) was used to trans-illumination screening of microvessels *in vivo*. Validation was performed using glass capillaries perfused with erythrocyte suspensions. Absorption spectra were recorded. For larger diameters (35-50µm) a wavelength range from 500nm to 600nm (green), and for small diameters (10-20µm) a range from 410nm to 440nm (blue) was used. Spectra for unknown SO_2 were compared to spectra for full-oxygenated and full-deoxygenated blood using a least square method. Results: In glass capillaries SO_2 values predicted by the microspectrophotometric method were close to data measured with a blood gas analyzer. In microvessels SO_2 levels for larger arterioles (35µm) and venules (50-60µm) of about 98% and 70%, respectively were estimated. Upon local deoxygenation by superfusion with Na-dithionite venular SO_2 levels fell to 0%. Conclusion: Imaging systems, which are widely used to assess functional parameters like e.g. intracellular Ca^{2+}- concentration, can be used to measure SO_2 levels during intravital microscopy. Supported by DFG (FOR341).

PAT 4

ARE LOCAL CHANGES IN BRAIN TEMPERATURE CORRELATED TO HEMODYNAMIC AND/OR METABOLIC EVENTS?

Mª.L. Luis-García, F.A. Martín, C. Merino, M.A. Castellano and J.L. González Mora*.
Dep. Fisiología. Fac. de Medicina. Univ. de La Laguna, Tenerife, 38007. Islas Canarias. Spain.

Although it is known that relatively large increases in local brain temperature can occur during behaviural studies and in response to enviromental stimuli, the source of this heat has not been cleary established. Some authors argue that hyperthermia produced after a stimulus is due to blood flow increase while other authors think that local hyperthermia is produced by the metabolic activity of the neurons, to clarify this issue, Sprague-Dawley rats were are anaesthetized for surgical procedures (Aproved by the Local Animal and Use Comitee) and local temperature, neurotransmitter realese (by *in vivo* voltametry), regional blood flow (by laser doppler flowmetry) and haemodynamic and metabolic parameters (by in vivo visible spectroscopy) were monitored bilateraly in rat striata after electrical stimulation of Middle forebrain bundle which induces a well known synaptical dopamine release in striatum. The results showed that after electrical stimulation, the local temperature increases in a very similar kinetic to DA release. Furthermore, changes in blood flow matched the temperature fluctuations and DA electrical evoked release. However, some results suggest that cerebral blood flow and temperature changes are not always connected, indicating complex relationships between metabolic and hemodinamic parameters and temperature. Bearing in mind that neural activity is accompanied by heat release, the local metabolic consequences of widely correlated neural activity appears to be the primary source of the increase in brain temperature even if changes in blood flow can also produce changes in brain temperature.

PAT 5

APPLICATION OF A DIGITAL DECONVOLUTION TECHNIQUE TO "IN VIVO" BRAIN TEMPERATURE MEASUREMENT AS AN INDEX OF METABOLIC REGULATION

C. Merino*, Mª.L. Luís-García, F.A. Martín, M.A. Castellano and J.L. González-Mora.
Dep. Fisiología. Fac. de Medicina. Univ. de La Laguna, Tenerife, 38007. Islas Canarias. Spain.

Many authors are investigating local temperature fluctuations in the brain; however the relationship between local temperature and other physiological parameters has never been established. Current temperature measurements are not completely accurate over time due to the physical constraints of the sensor, such as heat accumulation and dissipation. Thus, deconvolution techniques were evaluated for removing the sensor's own response to temperature changes and then trying to isolate local brain temperature fluctuations. Assuming linearity and time invariance of the sensor, the system's impulse response function was obtained via digital differentiation of the step response. Several digital differentiators were studied for this purpose. The step response of the system was obtained in different environments (including static air, water, air flow and different *in vivo* rat brain areas) by applying an infrared beam directly over the sensor through a micro optic fibre (100 μm ϕ). With this set-up we were able to reproduce the square pulse applied to the sensor using its output. The deconvolution technique developed was applied to simultaneous *in vivo* measurements of local temperature, blood-flow (Doppler flowmetry) and neurotransmitter release using in vivo amperometry with the aim of establishing their interrelationship. Deconvolution provides a method to obtain actual temperature changes, enabling further comparative kinetic studies of all those physiological parameters, contributing to clarify the exact mechanism that underlies neurovascular coupling.

PAT 6

CONFORMATIONAL CHANGES DURING FIBRINOGEN-LIGAND BINDING FOLLOWED BY FLUORESCENCE SPECTROSCPY

S. Gonçalves, N. C. Santos, J. Martins e Silva, C. Saldanha
Instituto de Bioquímica/ Faculdade de Medicina de Lisboa/ Unidade de Biopatologia Vascular/ Instituto de Medicina Molecular, 1649-028 Lisboa Portugal.

An unknown binding mechanism can relate increased erythrocyte aggregation with plasma fibrinogen concentration. Several studies have shown that an increase in fibrinogen levels is associated with the risk of cardiovascular disease and cerebrovascular disorders, infections, inflammations, trauma and to others factors such as hypertension and obesity. A previous *in vitro* study has shown an impaired erythrocyte aggregation in the presence of β-estradiol. The study of ligand binding to fibrinogen could provide information about the functionality of this protein during erythrocyte aggregation. Fluorescence spectroscopy experiments were performed in order to study fibrinogen-binding properties in the presence of different β-estradiol concentrations (1-77 nM). The fluorescence spectra did not show changes in the fluorescence emission wavelength maximum (λ = 344 nm). The protein shows diminished fluorescence intensities upon binding to β-estradiol. To evaluate the average accessibility of emissive tryptophans exposed during the fibrinogen-β estradiol binding, at different concentrations of the ligand, fluorescence-quenching experiments were performed using cesium, iodide and acrylamide (0.8 μM – 0.160 M). The quenching parameters obtained at different β-estradiol concentrations (0, 34 or 55 nM) show alterations that can be related with either possible conformational changes or a discrete reorganization of tryptophan residues during fibrinogen-ligand binding.

PBC 1

ROLE OF LECTIN-LIKE OXIDIZED LOW-DENSITY LIPOPROTEIN RECEPTOR-1 (LOX-1) ON ACTIVATED PLATELET ADHESION TO HUMAN BRAIN MICROVASCULAR ENDOTHERIAL CELLS UNDER FLOW IN VITRO

N. Tanahashi, Y. Itoh, M. Tomita, N. Suzuki
Department. of Neurology, Keio University, Tokyo 160-8582, Japan

Recently, lectin-like oxidized low density lipoprotein receptor-1 (LOX-1) was identified in endothelial cells and platelets. It was also found that negative phospholipids exposed on activation on the surface of platelets are epitopes for LOX-1. We examined the role of LOX-1 on activated platelet adhesion to human brain microvascular endothelial cells (HBEC).
HBECs were cultured on a coverglass and put in the observation chamber of video-enhanced contrast (VEC) microscopy. Platelet rich plasma (PRP) [N=6;control group], PRP containing ADP (2 μM) [N=7;ADP group] or PRP containing ADP (2 μM) and JTX92 (10 μg/ml; anti-human LOX-1 antibody) [N=5, anti-LOX-1 group] were superfused with an infusion pump at a low shear rate (10/sec) for 30 min and washed out. Interaction between platelets and HBEC was observed by VEC microscopy.
Platelet adhesion to HBEC was rarely seen in the control group. However, ADP-stimulated platelet adhered to HBEC. Anti-human LOX-1 antibody inhibited platelet adhesion. The average number of platelets adhering and aggregating to HBEC in each group was 0.3 ± 0.7/ 900 μm^2 in the control group, 22.3 ± 10.4/ 900 μm^2 in the ADP group (P<0.01, vs control), and 1.8 ± 2.5/ 900 μm^2 in the anti-LOX-1 group (p<0.01, vs ADP group), respectively. The above results showed anti-human LOX-1 antibody ameliorated platelet adhesion to HBEC at a low-flow state in vitro indicating that LOX-1 plays an important role in platelet adhesion to HBEC.

PBC 2

EFFECTS OF VELNACRINE MALEATE IN THE LEUKOCYTE-ENDOTHELIAL CELL INTERACTIONS IN RAT CREMASTER MICROCIRCULATORY NETWORK

A.S. Silva, C. Saldanha, J. Martins e Silva
Instituto de Bioquímica, Faculdade de Medicina de Lisboa, Unidade de Biopatologia Vascular, Instituto de Medicina Molecular
1649-028 Lisboa, Portugal

The expression of acetylcholinesterase (AChE) in proinflammatory cells has supported the hypothesis that this protein plays a role in intercellular adhesion, beyond its acetylcholine hydrolysis ability. Previous results of our group show that velnacrine (VM), an acetylcholinesterase inhibitor, increases the number of rolling leukocytes in post-capillary venules of Wistar rats' cremaster muscle. In order to evaluate the influence of the local application of velnacrine and acetylcoline (ACh), on the microcirculation in post-capillary venules of Wistar rats' cremaster muscle, the number of rolling leukocytes was monitorized. The number of adherent leukocytes, the diameter of the respective venule and the neighbouring arteriole were also determined. The results have shown that in presence of velnacrine there is significant increase of the rolling leukocytes (1.36±1.05 vs 1.96±1.15), as well as an increase of the adherent ones (1.04±1.03 vs 1.50±1.20). When ACh was also added the results obtained suggest that the effect of the velnacrine counters the one of acetylcholine, leading to the hypothesis that there is a specific interaction between velnacrine and acetylcholinesterase. The measurement of the venules and arterioles diameters allows us to conclude that acetylcholine induced vasodilatation either alone or in association with velnacrine. In opposition, in the venules, both efectors and velnacrine alone lead to vasoconstriction. We raise the hypothesis that the different vasoactive effects of VM and ACh on the venular and arteriolar sectors could be mediated by different signal transduction mechanism of AChE.

PBC 3

THE STUDY OF VELNACRINE MALEATE EFFECTS ON ERYTHROCYTES SECOND MESSENGERS

F.A.Carvalho, J. Martins-Silva, C. Saldanha
Instituto de Bioquímica, Faculdade de Medicina de Lisboa. Unidade de Biopatologia Vascular, Instituto de Medicina Molecular, 1649-028 Lisboa, Portugal.

Acetylcholine (ACh) has been detected in human blood. ACh receptors and acetylcholinesterase (AChE) are present in erythrocytes membranes. We tested the ACh effect on the nitric oxide production, the cAMP and cGMP concentration on erythrocytes suspensions, in absence or in presence of velnacrine maleate (VM, AChE inhibitor). We used human erythocytes suspensions in sodium chloride 0.9% pH 7 (haematocrit 0.05%) to measure the NO production with a amperometric NO sensor during stimulation with ACh 10 μM in absence or in presence of VM 10 μM. For quantification of the total cellular cAMP and cGMP we incubate the erythrocytes suspensions (haematocrit 45%), for 15 minutes at 37°C, with ACh (0, 0.01μM and 10 μM) in absence or in presence of VM 10 μM. After that we lysed them and used the supernatant for the enzyme immunoassay kits. We observed that ACh induce an increase on the erythrocytes NO production and the presence of VM reduced this increase (P=0.009, n=10). The erythrocytes ACh stimulation does not produced significant diferences in cAMP control levels and the presence of VM was also insignificant. Although cGMP levels increased with ACh and this fact is more relevant for low ACh concentrations. The VM significant decreased these levels and leads them to near the control values.
These results demonstrated that ACh modulate the NO and the cGMP production on erythrocytes and that this effect could be mediated by unknown interactions with the membrane enzyme acetylcholinesterase. The signal transduction mechanisms that leads to cAMP production seams not to be related or activated by the presence of ACh on erythrocytes.

PBC 4

GRAMICIDIN D, DITHIOTHREITOL AND CYTOCHALASIN B EFFECTS ON ERYTHROCYTE EXOVESICULATION

N. C. Santos, J. Martins e Silva, C. Saldanha
Instituto de Bioquímica/ Faculdade de Medicina de Lisboa/ Unidade de Biopatologia Vascular/ Instituto de Medicina Molecular, 1649-028 Lisboa Portugal.

The use of diphenylhexatriene (DPH), trimethylamino-diphenylhexatriene (TMA-DPH) or heptadecyl-hydroxycoumarin (C_{17}-HC) allows to, simultaneously and with the same molecule, to induce erythrocyte exovesiculation and label the released vesicles with the fluorescent probe. This method was used to evaluate gramicidin D (a channel-forming peptide), dithiothreitol (a reducing agent) and cytochalasin B (a toxin that disrupts contractile microfilaments) effects on the human erythrocytes vesiculation process. The release of cholesterol and phospholipids in exovesicles at longer incubation times was only detectable in the presence of these effectors. When C_{17}-HC was used to induce the vesiculation, the presence of gramicidin or dithiothreitol lead to a drastic decrease on the [Phospholipids]/[Cholesterol] ratio. However, in the samples with dithiothreitol, this variation did not result in the expectable decrease of membrane fluidity. These effects can be related with the presence of lipid rafts, the transbilayer lipids reorientation induced by gramicidin or dithiothreitol, and the cholesterol-dependent gramicidin channels inactivation. At most of the experimental conditions under evaluation, cytochalasin B induced significantly increased cholesterol concentration and acetylcholinesterase (AChE) enzyme activity on the released vesicles.

PCM 1

HYALURONIDASE REDUCES CORONARY GLYCOCALYX VOLUME IN GOATS

J. Brands, J.W.G.E. Van Teeffelen, E.P. Baerends, J.A.E. Spaan, H. Vink
Medical Physics, Academic Medical Center, Meibergdreef 15, Amsterdam, NL 1105 AZ, The Netherlands

A 0.5 μm thick glycocalyx covers the luminal side of striated muscle capillaries (Vink & Duling, 1996). The layer is freely accessible to neutral (texas red labeled) dextrans of MW 40 kD (D40) but excludes flowing red blood cells and large anionic (fluorescein isothiocyanate labeled) dextrans of 70 kD (D70) and limits perfused capillary volume.

In open-chest anesthetized goats, D40 and D70 were simultaneously infused via a perfusion system into the left main artery for 2 min, and 1 ml samples collected from the coronary sinus every 2.5 s. Outflow concentration curves of D40 and D70 were constructed and coronary glycocalyx volume (Vg) calculated from the amount of D40 permeating into the glycocalyx and its steady-state concenctration.

In control, Vg was 2.1 ± 0.6 ml/100 g (n=7, P<0.05). Degradation of intravascular hyaluronan (hyaluronidase; 25 U/ml for 45 min) decreased Vg to –0.2 ± 0.7 ml/100 g (n=5, NS). Given a perfused coronary capillary volume of 10 ml/100 g Left Ventricle (Van der Ploeg et al., 1993) and a LV to whole heart weight of 60%, our data indicate that the glycocalyx occupies 23 ± 6 % of coronary capillary volume. At a perfusion pressure of 110 mmHg, hyaluronidase increased baseline coronary blood flow from 92 ± 13 to 138 ± 20 ml/min/100 g (P<0.05), indicating that modulation of glycocalyx volume and/or permeability has the potential to affect coronary flow. Support: NWO (902-16-192), KNAW (to HV), NHS (96.120 JvT, 2003B181 JB).

PCM 2

PRESSURE-DEPENDENT INWARD REMODELING IN ISOLATED SUB-ENDOCARDIAL ARTERIOLES IS PREVENTED BY CALCIUM BLOCKADE

O. Sorop; E.N.T.P. Bakker; J.A.E. Spaan, and E. VanBavel
Dept. of Medical Physics, University of Amsterdam
Academic Medical Center, Meibergdreef 9, 1105AZ,
PO Box 22700, 1100 DE Amsterdam, The Netherlands

Due to the contracting surrounding myocardium large variations of transvascular pressure exist in sub-endocardial arterioles. Coronary stenosis affects these pressure profiles. We hypothesized that altered transvascular pressure profiles affect tone and structure of sub-endocardial arterioles, and that maintained pharmacological vasodilation induces outward remodeling under these conditions. 36 isolated porcine sub-endocardial vessels were cannulated and cultured for 3 days. Vessels were subjected to different transvascular pressure profiles: *Osc 80*: mean 80 mmHg, 60 mmHg peak-peak sine wave pulsation amplitude at 1.5 Hz; *St 80*: steady 80 mmHg; *Osc 40*: mean 40 mmHg, 30 mmHg amplitude; *St 40*: steady 40 mmHg. Under the *Osc 80* profile, modest tone developed, reducing the diameter to 69.5±13.6% of the maximal, passive diameter. No inward remodeling was found here, as judged from the passive pressure-diameter relation after 3 days of culture. Under all other profiles, much deeper tone developed (e.g. *Osc 40*: 21.4±3.4%). In addition, these vessels showed eutrophic inward remodeling (e.g. *Osc 40*: passive diameter reduction by 26.3±1.6%). The calcium blocker, amlodipine induced maintained dilation in *St 40* vessels, and reversed the 23.4±2.5% inward remodeling to 13.4±3.6% outward remodeling towards day 3.
Conclusions: During obstructive coronary artery disease, microvascular mean pressure and pulsation amplitude may both be reduced. Our data indicate that either condition leads to microvascular constriction followed by inward remodeling. These effects could be reversed by amlodipine.

PCV 1

VICIOUS CIRCLE BETWEEN CEREBRAL MICROCIRCULATION AND LIPID PEROXIDATION DURING STROKE

N.Bolokadze, G.Mchedlishvili, N.Momtselidze, R. Solomonia Microcírculation Research Center and Laboratory of Biochemical Neuropharmacology, Beritashvili Institute of Physiology, 14 Gotua 8tr., o 160, Tbilis Georgia

The aim of the present study was investigation of the relationship of the microhemorheological properties and lipid peroxidation during cerebral stroke in the damaged hemisphere. The studies were carried out on 26 patients, suffering from critically deteriorated stroke. As a control we analysed 7 patients without evidence of brain tissue damage. Blood samples were drawn from the homolateral internal jugular vein. The patients gave their consent to the investigation according to the principles of the Declaration of Helsinki. For the "in vitro" studies blood samples were taken ftom the cubital veins of 15 healthy subjects and incubated with: MDA at final concentration of 2 and 4 µmoles for one hour at 37°C. RBC aggregation was evaluated by using the "Georgian technique". MDA was determined by colour reaction with N-methyl-2-phenylin-dole at 45°C. In blood flowing out ftom the damaged hemisphere the RBC aggregation was by almost 80% higher (P<0.005) and MDA amount was by 55% higher (P<0.05) as compared to the blood flowing out ftom the corresponding hemisphere of control patients. In the in vitro conditions RBC aggregation was increased in the groups treated with MDA as compared to the control group: by 80 % (P<O.OOI, MDA fInal concentration 2 µmoles) and by 120% (P<O.OO 1, MDA final Concentration 4 µmoles). The results indicate that during cerebral stroke both microcirculation and tissue metabolism are deteriorated and these two processes are closely interrelated. Therefore a vicious circle is created in the damaged hemisphere where lipid peroxidation and blood rheological properties are interdependent.

PCV 2

TIME-DEPENDENT AMYGDALOALLOCORTICAL NEURO-ENDOTHELIAL COX-2, TNF-ALPHA, IL-1BETA EXPRESSION, EDEMA AND MICROHEMORRHAGES FORMATION INDUCED BY GENERALIZED CONVULSIVE SEIZURES IN THE RAT.

A. Régnier, Y. Calando, E. Vicaut and S. Mraovitch.
Laboratoire d'Etude de la Microcirculation, Université ParisVII, 10 avenue de Verdun 75010 Paris, France.

We recently demonstrated that generalized convulsive seizures (GCS), induced by cholinergic stimulation of the thalamus, provoke a focal amygdaloallocortical infarction characterized by COX-2 inhibition, TNF-alpha and IL-1beta induction followed by edema with microhemorrhages. Here, we determined the temporal progression and anatomical specificity of the inflammatory processes leading to edema and microhemorrhages. Adult Wistar rats were injected stereotaxically with carbachol under anesthesia. Behavioral alterations were observed for 2h. After at least one episode of GCS, animals were sacrificed at 3h, 6h, 12h, 24h, 48h and 72h. Immunohistochemically processed sections were examined with a camera lucida. Edema and microhemorrhage sites were estimated on digital photographs of fresh frozen tissue using an image analyzer. From 2h to 72h, the inhibition of neuronal COX-2 expression included the piriform cortex, the amygdala (except lateral nucleus) and the entorhinal cortex. Endothelial cytokine expression appeared at 3h and 6h in the piriform cortex and the basolateral amygdala, extending to the insular cortex at 12h and 24h, and to all nuclei of the amygdala between at 48-72h, except the cortical nucleus. Edema associated with microhemorrhages was observed along the amygdalloallocortical axis from 24h for up to 72h. The number of microhemorrhagic transformation sites increased up to 72h. We conclude that GCS initially induce specific regional and temporal neuroendothelial injuries leading to delayed edema with microhemorrhagic transformations.

PCV 3

IBUPROFEN MODULATES THE AMYGDALOALLOCORTICAL ENDOTHELIAL INFLAMMATION AND EDEMA INDUCED BY GENERALIZED CONVULSIVE SEIZURES IN THE RAT.

A. Régnier, E. Vicaut and S. Mraovitch.
Laboratoire d'Etude de la Microcirculation, Université ParisVII, 10 avenue de Verdun 75010 Paris, France.

Generalized convulsive seizures (GCS) induced by cholinergic stimulation of the thalamus, provoke a focal amygdaloallocortical infarction characterized by neuronal COX-2 inhibition, endothelial TNF-alpha and IL-1beta induction followed by edema with microhemorrhages. We sought to determine whether this cascade of events may be modulated by ibuprofen. Adult Wistar rats were injected stereotaxically with carbachol under anesthesia in the unilateral lateral thalamus. Ibuprofen was injected i.p. (20mg/Kg) either 30min or 6h after the first episode of GCS. COX-2, TNF-alpha and IL-1beta immunohistochemistry were processed and edema and microhemorrhage sites were estimated on digital photographs. The early injection of ibuprofen (n=3) suppressed the inhibition of neuronal COX-2 expression. The endothelial cytokines expression was increased. In contrast, the delayed ibuprofen injection (n=3) potentiated the inhibition of neuronal COX-2 and the induction of endothelial TNF-alpha and IL-1beta expression. In untreated epileptic rats (n=5), edema, associated with sporadic microhemorrhages, ranged between 6±0.2% and 11±0.1% with the maximal surface area at the level of the amygdala. The early injection of ibuprofen, caused a marked increase in edema (n=4) reaching 23±0.6% in the posterior amygdalo-allocortical area and, microhemorrhagic sites increased in number. The delayed injection of ibuprofen provoked a dramatic decrease in the edema surface area, 5±0.2% in the posterior amygdaloallocortical area and, microhemorrhagic sites were absent. We conclude that ibuprofen has time-dependent effect on COX-2, cytokines expression and consequently on edema and microhemorrhages.

PDM 1

CAPILLARY BLOOD FLOW AND CAPILLARY BLOOD SUGAR IN FINGERS AND TOES OF PATIENTS WITH TYPE II DIABETES MELLITUS

Michael Azziz, Mona El Amir, Mohammed Sheta and Aly el Ashmaui
From the department of Medicine, Cairo University, Egypt

The study was performed on 20 non insulin dependant diabetes mellitus free of vascular complications or neuropathy of the foot and 10 patients with diabetic foot in addition to 10 age matched control group.It was found that the capillary flow in fingers with complicated diabetic patients had lower basal value, and prolonged time to peak time on thermal stimulation when compared to fingers in studies in uncomplicated diabetics, on the other hand, more pronounced changes were detected in the toes, where toes in patients with vascular complications where found to have marked diminution of basal flow, prolongation of time to peak and significant decrease in the percent change after thermal stimulation. On the other hand, the basal flux as well as the % change was found to be diminished in the toes as compared to the fingers. No significant difference regarding capillary blood sugar between obtained from the finger and toes in control group. No difference of statistical significance was found between the fingers of uncomplicated and complicated diabetics regarding the capillary sugar as well as between the toes of uncomplicated and complicated diabetics. Capillary blood sugar were found to be higher in toes of complicated diabetic compared to their fingers, the same was true regarding the uncomplicated group. However, toes with complicated diabetes had more pronounced changes in the Laser Doppler flow when compared to fingers in the form of lower basal flow, diminished % changes and prolongation of time to peak, while toes of uncomplicated diabetics have less defect compared to the corresponding fingers. It was concluded that the resistance of the uptake of glucose at the cellular level might be selective (toe more than fingers). This might be associated with more pronounced endothelial dysfunction.

PDM 2

ENDOTHELIAL DYSFUNCTION AND MICROANGIOPATHIC CHANGES IN FIRST DEGREE RELATIVES OF PATIENTS WITH TYPE 2 DIABETES ASSESSED BY IONTOPHORESIS

Mona Ali Nashaat ,Aly El-Ashmaoui, , and Hoda Abd El-Ghany*, departments of Internal Medicine and Clinical Pathology* , Cairo University, Egypt

Endothelial function was studied in two groups with age and sex matched subjects: 14 normoglycemic normotensive first degree relative of patients with type 2 diabetes and ten non-smoker normal subjects taken as controls. Laser Doppler perfusion imaging was used to measure vasodilatation in the foot skin in response to iontophoresis of 1% acetylcholine. In the same time, maximal skin microvascular vasodilatation in response to heat was performed. Peak response of skin blood flow due to dilatation effect induced by iontophoretically acetylcholine in 20sec, 40sec and 80sec was found to be significantly reduced in relatives of type 2 diabetes compared to controls. Baseline to peak flow readings (% change) for microcirculation of the foot are still significantly reduced in first degree relatives of type 2 diabetes in response to iontophoresis by acetylcholine. The difference in flow associated endothelium dependent vasodilatation could not be attributed to other variables, because the study could not show any difference in relation to age, sex or BMIs. The maximum blood flow as measured by Laser Doppler fluximetry (LDF) in response to heat was found to be some what lower in the first degree relatives of patients with type 2 diabetes but results was not of statistical significance and the difference between patients and controls was not marked. These results suggest that abnormalities in endothelial function are present early in individuals at risk of developing type 2 diabetes, well before any clinical symptoms are present, even at euglycemic stage.

PDM 3

MICROCIRCULATORY EVALUATION OF NON DIABETIC SUBJECTS WITH STRONG FAMILY HISTORY OF TYPE II DIABETES.

Mona Ali Nashaat, Aly El-Ashmaoui, and Fatma El-Mongy.* Departments of Internal medicine and Clinical pathology*Faculty of Medicine, Cairo University, Egypt

The study was performed on thirty five patients with type 2 diabetes mellitus (twenty non smoker with no vascular complications and fifteen patients with no vascular complications). Twenty non smoker diabetic offspring were included. Twenty normal subjects were chosen in 2 age groups (20-40 years and another group 40-60 years) to match for the older diabetic patients and young diabetic offspring. A significant decrease in basal skin blood flow in the diabetic patients as well as in the diabetic offspring subjects was detected. Furthermore, a significant increase in time taken by the diabetic subjects to show reactive hyperemia compared to controls. This delay in time was not observed in the diabetic offspring. The absolute values of maximum hyperemia shows profound depression that was significantly lower in the diabetic patients with and without vascular complications compared to controls. A decrease in the maximum hyperemic response was also noticed in the diabetic offspring group compared to controls. The percent change showed significant difference in the group of the diabetics with vascular complications compared to the controls. A significant difference in LDF results in patients with and without microalbuminuria, neuropathy and retinopathy in the diabetic patients. Significant inverse correlations were found between vascular reactivity and fasting plasma glucose and LDL, while a direct correlation was found with HDL cholesterol. It was concluded that , an endothelial inhereted defect might be present long before the appearance of the metabolic and the clinical syndrome of type II diabetes.

PDM 4

MICROVASCULAR CHANGES IN DIABETIC ULCERS

Dina Shaheen, Mohammed Sharaf, Aly El Ashmaoui and Sherif El Hawary, Department of Medicine, Cairo University, Egypt

The aim of the present work is to evaluate the microcirculation function in diabetic ulcers in an attempt to study the pathogenesis which could help in planning the management.
Material and methods: patients were divided into 3 groups :
Group I NIDDM with diabetic ulcers (17 patients).
Group II: 10 NIDDM with no ulcers.
Group III: 10 normal age matched healthy control.
Group IV : 9 patients with traumatic ulcers.
All Patients were subjected to Laser Doppler flowmetry and transcutaneous O_2 determination.
Mean basal laser flowmetry was found to diminished in diabetics with ulcers compared to diabetic with no ulcers or to traumatic cases.
Transcutaneous O_2 was found to be diminished in diabetics with ulcers compared to control group. However no significant changes was found when compared to diabetic with no ulcers or to traumatic cases. Diabetic foot with no ulcers have diminished but not significant $tcpO_2$ value when compared to control group.
Furthermore, the power of vasomotion was found to be diminished in diabetics with ulcers when compared to diabetics with no ulcers and to traumatic cases.
No difference of statistical importance was found regarding the frequency of vasomotion.
These findings point to exaggeration of the diminished $tcpO_2$ in diabetic foot the diminished basal flow and power of vasomotion observed in diabetic ulcers could be a primary or secondary effect and need further study.

PDM 5

POSSIBLE ROLE OF ENDOTHELIN I IN THE PATHOGENESIS MICROVASCULAR COMPLICATIONS IN TYPE II DIABETES MELLITUS

Rania Meawad, Mona Nashaat, Aly El Ashmaoui and Hoda Abdel Ghany
From the Department of Medicine and Clinical Pathology, Cairo University, Egypt

Thirty patients with type II diabetes mellitus were selected. Exclusion criteria included: patients with cardiac affection including coronary artery disease, patients with pulmonary disease, renal failure and patients with peripheral arterial disease.They were further divided into 20 patients without neuropathy, retinopathy or nephropathy and 10 patients having any of these complications either single or combined. These cases were compared to the following groups:10 age matched non diabetic healthy, non smoker control subjects, 10 young healthy subjects (below the age of 18 years) with both diabetic parents. 6 young age matched to the previous group with no family history of diabetes mellitus. All patients were subjected to Laser Doppler flowmetry, and endothelin I estimation. Diabetic patients in general whether with or without complications were found to have elevated level of endothelin I compared to age matched control subjects (18.8 +/- 7.9 for patients without complications , 19.21 +/- 12 in patients with complications compared to 2.58 +/- 1.1 in non diabetic subjects, p<0.001). This was coupled with statistically significant drop of percent increase of Laser Doppler flowmetry after thermal stimulation in diabetic with complications as compared with control subjects. Endothelin I was specifically higher in diabetes with retinopathy as compared to those without retinopathy. Children's with family history of diabetes mellitus were found to have higher level of endothelin I as compared to age matched control (16.6 +/- 3.5 and 8.7 +/- 2.2 respectively , p<0.001) and diminished % change to thermal stimulation compared to age matched control. It was concluded that endothelin I might play an important role in the pathogenesis of microvascular complications in type II diabetes.

PDM 6

HOW INSULINEMIA INFLUENCES SKIN MICROCIRCULATION OF LOWER LIMBS IN HEALTHY SUBJECTS.

Krcma M., Jankovec Z., Lacigova S., Zourek M., Mudra J., Rusavy Z.
Diabetologic Center, 1st Department of Internal Medicine, University Hospital, Plzen, 32300, Czech Republic

Objective: Recent papers describe insulin-mediated vasodilatation. The question, if it is only vasodilatation caused by increased glucose uptake or solitary insuline effect, is not satisfactorily answered. Our aim was to examine skin perfusion in dependency on insulinemia in healthy subjects.

Research design and methods: All volunteers were informed in detail about the procedures and signed informed consent. The protocol of this study was approved by ethical committee. In our study a two-stage hyperinsulinemic euglycaemic clamp was performed, with insulinemia 100 and 250 mIU/ml and glycaemia 5,0 mmol/l (3% standard deviation). Before the clamp and in steady states, microcirculation was measured by Laser-Doppler flowmetry and transcutaneous oximetry and energy expenditure was measured by indirect calorimetry. Results (average and standard deviation) were evaluated with paired t-test.

Results: Lower limb skin perfusion, measured by laser Doppler, was at basal conditions (1456 ± 841) %, and increased at lower hyperinsulinemia (100m IU/l) to (1632 ± 894) %, and at higher hyperinsulinemia (250m IU/l) to (1867 ± 1026) %. Both results were statistically significant ($p < 0.05$). Post occlusive hyperemia test showed significantly increased perfusion ($p < 0.001$) at lower insulinemia 1,7s in comparison with 5,2s at basal conditions, at higher insulinemia 1,4s.

Conclusions: Post occlusive hyperemia test in accordance with heating test showed significantly increasing skin perfusion in the course of artificial hyperinsulinemia, dependency on the dose was not statistically significant. Presented results will be used for comparison with diabetic patients with and without neuropathy.

PDM 7

PPARg ACTIVATION BY REDUCING OXIDATIVE STRESS PROTECTS MICROVASCULAR FUNCTION IN TYPE 2 DIABETES MELLITUS

Z Bagi, G Kaley, A Koller
Dept. of Physiology, New York Medical Coll., Valhalla, NY 10595, USA
Dept. of Pathophysiology, Semmelweis University, Budapest, Hungary

Type 2 diabetes mellitus (T-2-DM) is accompanied by increased vascular oxidative stress. Although, agonists of peroxisome proliferator-activated receptor gamma (PPARγ) have been shown to have beneficial effects primarily on metabolic disorders, we hypothesized that they also improve microvascular function by reducing oxidative stress, via a mechanism that is unrelated to their effect on hyperglycemia and hyperinsulinemia. Control and T-2-DM mice (C57BL/KsJ-db-/db-) were treated with rosiglitazone (ROSI, 3 mg/kg/day) for 7 days, which did not significantly affect serum concentrations of glucose and insulin. In db/db mice, compared to controls, serum levels of 8-isoprostane (a marker of *in vivo* oxidative stress) and dihydroethydine-detectable superoxide production in carotid arteries were significantly elevated, which were reduced by ROSI treatment. Coronary arterioles (~ 80 μm), isolated from db/db mice, exhibited reduced dilations to acetylcholine, NO-donor (NONOate) and flow that were restored either by application of superoxide dismutase (SOD) or by ROSI treatment. Gracilis muscle arterioles (~ 90 μm) of db/db mice exhibited an increased pressure-induced basal tone (from 20 to 120 mmHg), which was reduced by administration of catalase or by ROSI treatment. In aorta of db/db mice, activities of SOD and catalase were reduced, whereas NAD(P)H-oxidase activity was enhanced. ROSI treatment enhanced catalase and reduced NAD(P)H-oxidase activity, but did not affect the activity of SOD. These findings suggest that in type 2 diabetic mice ROSI treatment reduces the level of vascular NAD(P)H-oxidase-derived superoxide and hydrogen peroxide. Thus, in addition to the previously revealed beneficial metabolic effects, the antioxidant action of PPARγ agonists may protect microvascular function in type 2 diabetes mellitus.

(Supported by Hungarian OTKA T-034779, NHLBI HL-46813, HL-43023)

PDM 8

IS MAXIMUM BLOOD FLOW IN CHILDREN WITH DIABETES PREDICTIVE OF LATER MICROVASCULAR COMPLICATIONS?

A.C.Shore, K.F.Mills, K.Price, J.Tripp, K.M.MacLoed, J.E.Tooke.
Institute of Biomedical and Clinical Science, Peninsula Medical School, Barrack Road, Exeter, EX2 5AX, Uk

Microalbuminuria in type 1 diabetes is an established risk factor for renal disease progression and the earliest clinical sign of diabetic nephropathy.

Previous studies in children with diabetes have indicated that functional abnormalities of the microcirculation occur in the absence of clinically detectable microalbuminuria. The aim of this study was to determine whether early microvascular dysfunction was predictive of later microvascular complications. 73 children with type 1 diabetes completed microvascular testing, 40 of whom had follow up information available. 25 were complication free and 15 had either microalbuminuria (9), retinopathy (5) or both (1). The adults who have developed complications had significantly lower maximum hyperaemia (MH) as children (1.07V vs 1.52V,p=0.001,t-test). Although their duration of diabetes at the time of testing was significantly higher in the group with complications (6.3 vs 2.7years, p=0.0001), the reduction in MH was greater than that expected from duration alone. Follow up time, age and glycated haemoglobin at the time of testing were not significantly different. This has potential implications for clinical care, in that it suggests that MH may be a useful clinical tool in predicting complications before the development of microalbuminuria and clinically significant neuropathy.

PEB 1

ACTIVATION OF NF-kB BY REACTIVE OXYGEN SPECIES MEDIATES INDUCTION OF PAI-1 EXPRESSION IN VASCULAR ENDOTHELIAL CELLS

Maria Swiatkowska[*1], Janusz Szemraj[*2], Jolanta Niewiarowska[*1], and James K. Liao
Cardiovascular Division, Brigham & Women's Hospital and Harvard Medical School, Boston, Massachusetts 02115, USA. [*]Department of Molecular and Medical Biophysics, [1]Department of Biochemistry, [2]Medical University of Lodz, Lodz, Poland

Objective: Plasminogen activator inhibitor (PAI)-1 is an important physiological regulator of vascular hemostasis. PAI-1 is an acute phase reactant, which is induced by many pro-inflammatory and pro-oxidant factors such as TNFα and TGF-β1. We hypothesize that reactive oxygen species mediates TNFα-induced PAI-1 expression. **Methods**: Human endothelial cells were treated with TNFα or hydrogen peroxide with or without antioxidants, and intracellular superoxide anion production and oxidative stress were determined by lucigenin chemiluminescence and 2',7'-dichlorofluroscein (DCF) fluorescence, respectively. PAI-1 mRNA expression was determined by Northern blotting. PAI-1 gene transcription was determined by transfection of a PAI-1 promoter linked to a luciferase reporter. NF-κB activity was determined by electrophoretic mobility shift assay. Results: Treatment of endothelial cells with TNFα increased the generation of superoxide anion and oxidative stress. This corresponded to increase in PAI-1 mRNA expression, which was blocked by the antioxidant, N-acetylcysteine (NAC) and by overexpression of a super-suppressor phosphorylation-resistant IκBα.Indeed, TNFα stimulated NF-κB activity, which was inhibited by NAC. **Conclusion**: These findings indicate that NF-κB is an important regulator of TNFα-induced PAI-1 expression, and suggest that reactive oxygen species mediates PAI-1 expression via activation of NF-κB.

PEB 2

REGULATION OF EXPRESSION AND NEW ROLES FOR INTERCELLULAR ADHESION MOLECULE-2 (ICAM-2) IN ENDOTHELIAL CELL HOMEOSTASIS

M-T. Huang, J.C.Mason, E. Lidington, D.O.Haskard, A.M.Randi
BHF Cardiovascular Medicine, Eric Bywaters Centre, Hammersmith Hospital, Imperial College London, London W12 0NN, United Kingdom

Previously we reported that TNFα down-regulates the expression of the adhesion molecule ICAM-2 on human umbilical vein endothelial cells (HUVEC) through suppression of the transcription factor Erg, a member of the Ets family (McLaughlin F et al. J. Cell Sci 1999; 112: 4695-4703). Here we present new findings on the regulation of ICAM-2 expression and its novel role in endothelial cell homeostasis.

Objective: To investigate the regulation of ICAM-2 expression on endothelial cells and the role of ICAM-2 in endothelial homeostasis. **Method**: HUVEC were isolated by standard procedures. Murine cardiac endothelial cells (MCEC) were isolated from both control and ICAM-2 knockout (KO) mice by using positive selection with anti-endoglin magnetic beads. Flow cytometry and real-time PCR were used for surface protein and mRNA detection. **Summary of results**: 1) Expression of ICAM-2 on HUVEC was positively regulated by cell-cell contact at both protein and mRNA levels; 2) Up-regulation of ICAM-2 on HUVEC by cell contact correlated with increased Erg mRNA expression; 3) Expression of ICAM-2 on HUVEC was down-regulated by basic fibroblast growth factor and up-regulated by angiopoietin 1 at both protein and mRNA levels; 4) Using MCEC from ICAM-2 KO mice, we found that endothelial cell proliferation was not dependent on ICAM-2; however, the lack of ICAM-2 expression rendered endothelial cells vulnerable to apoptosis.

Conclusions: Our findings show that ICAM-2 plays a role in endothelial survival and is regulated during junction formation, suggesting its participation in endothelial homeostasis.

PEB 3

COMBINATION OF THE PERMEABILIZING EFFECTS OF VEGF AND HGF REDUCES BRAIN ENDOTHELIAL PERMEABILITY IN VITRO.

K. Voigt, J. Kraus, M. Clauss
Department of Neurology, University Hospital Giessen, D-35385 Giessen, Germany
MPI for Physiological and Clinical Research, D-61231 Bad Nauheim, Germany

Objective: VEGF promotes the permeability of the blood-brain barrier, possibly through induction of endothelial permeability. HGF increases paracellular permeability in human vascular endothelial cells. We examined whether exposure of a monolayer of brain endothelioma cells to both factors increases endothelial permeability in vitro.

Methods: The immortalized endothelioma cell line bEnd5 from mouse brain capillaries was grown to confluence for three weeks on semipermeable filters precoated with rat tail collagen. Culture media was replaced with Ringer-HEPES solution, and the paracellular permeability of radioactive [^{14}C]-sucrose and [^{3}H]-inulin across the endothelioma monolayers was determined after exposure to 40ng/ml VEGF or to 5μg/ml HGF for 3 hours before the assay, or to both. Permeability was compared to unstimulated controls, respectively.

Results: Exposure to VEGF or HGF alone lead to a significant increase of the permeability of the bEnd5 cells; this was less pronounced for HGF than VEGF. However, the combination of VEGF and HGF did not increase endothelial permeability significantly, as compared to unstimulated controls.

Conclusion: The results indicate that the combination of VEGF and HGF relieves their individual permeabilizing effects in the mouse brain endothelial cell line bEnd5. Therefore, VEGF and HGF may have interactive effects in these cells in vitro.

PEB 4

ACTIVATION OF NOTCH 1 INHIBITS PROLIFERATION IN HUMAN UMBILICAL VEIN ENDOTHELIAL CELLS (HUVECS)

N. Sulaiman, L. Leach, P.M. Wigmore
School of Biomedical Sciences, Queen's Medical Centre, Nottingham, NG7 2UH, UK.

Notch signalling is highly conserved throughout evolution and plays a fundamental role in determining cell fate during development. Depending on the cellular context, Notch signalling has been found to inhibit or induce, differentiation, proliferation and cell survival. We have studied the effect of Notch signalling on the proliferation of HUVECs. Umbilical cords were obtained with informed patient consent and ethical approval and HUVECs isolated by standard protocols. The optimum conditions for square wave electroporation of HUVECs were determined by transfecting the cells with an Enhanced Green Fluorescent Protein (GFP) plasmid. Using the conditions for GFP transfection, HUVECs were then transfected with an epitope-tagged intracellular domain of Notch1. Cells were pulse labelled with 5-bromo-2-deoxyuridine (BrdU) 24 hours after transfection. Immunofluorescent staining was used to detect the transfected cells, using an antibody to the epitope tag and proliferating cells using an anti-BrdU antibody. The optimum condition of HUVECs transfection are a single pulse of 210V and 50ms length. Using these conditions a transfection efficiency of 40% was achieved. Transfection of HUVECs with NICD plasmid resulted in a significant reduction in the number of BrdU positive cells compared with that of controls (51% vs 27.8%, $p<0.05$). This suggests that Notch signalling might induce a cell cycle arrest, probably in G1, which would be required for cell differentiation.

PEB 5

SIGNAL TRANSDUCTION PATHWAYS IN WALL SHEAR STRESS-REGULATED ENDOTHELIAL GENEXPRESSION

A. Zakrzewicz, A. Alter, W. Wunderlich, J. Abraham, M. Bongrazio and A. R. Pries
Department of Physiology, Charité Campus Benjamin Franklin, Berlin, 14195, Germany

Remodelling of microvascular networks occurs in response to altered blood flow conditions. A main mechanism of this response may be wall shear stress regulated genexpression in endothelial cells. In this study, we looked for shear stress-regulated genes and the signaltransduction pathways which mediate this generegulation.

Endothelial cells were isolated from human umbilical veins and exposed to defined laminar flow (6 dyn/cm^2, 24 h) using a cone-and-plate device. The involvement of signaltransduction pathways was tested with a pathway-specific genearray. Expression of flow-regulated endothelial genes was analysed by quantitative real-time RT-PCR with or without the presence of specific signal pathways inhibitors. Inactive analogues of these inhibitors served as negative controls.

Three pathways were significantly involved in long time (24 h) mechanotransduction: the PLC-pathway, the NFκB-, and the p53 system. Shear stress-dependent induction of Tie-2, METH-1, and Properdin was significantly reduced by inhibition of PLCγ, whereas none of the pathways tested seems to be involved in shear stress-dependent suppression of Angiopoietin-2, TSP-1 od CD36.

Thus, the PLC-pathway seems to be a main mediator for long lasting shear stress-regulated induction of endothelial genes. By contrast, at least in this study, we could not find so far a signal pathway for shear stress-regulated suppression of endothelial genes.

PEB 6

THE ANGIOGENIC SPROUTING RESPONSE TO COLLAGEN REQUIRES SRC FAMILY KINASE ACTIVITY.

J. F. Dye, M. Barnett, C. Linge & R. Sanders
RAFT Institute, Mount Vernon Hospital, Northwood, London HA6 2RN UK

Exposure of human placental microvascular endothelial cells (HPMEC) to collagen stimulates loss of cell-cell adhesion, angiogenic sprouting and migration, whereas laminin stimulates tubulogenesis. These responses are mediated by distinct integrins. We hypothesised that src family kinases (SFK) are required for responses to collagen, via integrin $\alpha 2\beta 1$.

Human term placentae were obtained with consent to establish HPMEC cultures from chorionic villus capillary fragments. Confluent cultures in microwells, in minimal medium or with the SFK inhibitor PP2 (50-800nM), were overlaid with gelling solutions of collagen or Matrigel and fixed after 48hr. 100 nM siRNA oligos to pp60c-src or p59-fyn or GAPDH were transfected into cells with lipofectamine2000 24hr prior to gel overlay. Expression was assessed by western blotting. Phospho-src levels were determined by western blotting and localised by immunofluorescence microscopy. Experiments were repeated with at least 3 cell isolates.

Inhibition of SFK activity by PP2, and siRNA to both c-src and fyn, abrogated monolayer disruption and angiogenic sprout responses to collagen, but had little effect on Matrigel-stimulated tube formation. Phospho-src levels in HPMEC were increased in response to collagen but decreased in response to matrigel. Phospho-src was immunolocalised to large focal adhesions in cells interacting with collagen. These were absent in the tube structures formed in Matrigel.

These results indicate that SFK activity is activated via $\alpha 2$ but not $\alpha 6$ integrins and is required for sprouting/migration and may be pivotal in regulating angiogenic morphology of HPMEC. We conclude that specific matrix-integrin signals represent a novel mechanism for regulating angiogenesic behaviour. Supported by the Dunhill Trust.

PEB 7

SIGNALLING PATHWAYS INVOLVED IN LYSOPHOSPHATIDYLCHOLINE INDUCED PHOSPHOLIPASE D ACTIVATION IN HUMAN ENDOTHELIAL CELLS.

S.McHarg, A.C.Shore, J.L.Whatmore
Institute of Biomedical and Clinical Sciences, Peninsula Medical School, Barrack Road, Exeter, EX2 5EQ, UK

Lysophosphatidylcholine (LPC) is a major component of oxidized LDL, and is implicated in atherogenesis. The signalling enzyme phospholipase D (PLD) is also implicated in the development of vascular disease, and has been reported to be activated by LPC in mammalian cells. However, the signalling pathways involved are not fully understood.

The aim of this study was to examine the involvement of tyrosine kinases (TK) and MAP kinases (MAPK) in LPC induced PLD activation in human endothelial cells.

Human umbilical vein endothelial cells (HUVECs) were isolated from umbilical cords by collagenase digestion, and used at passage 3. [^{3}H] myristic acid labelled HUVECs were treated with 20µm LPC and varying doses of TK or MAPK inhibitors. PLD activity was assessed by quantitation of ^{3}H phosphatidylethanol.

20µm LPC evoked a significant increase in PLD activation, with a mean increase of 385±281% (control=100%) (n=32, $p<0.001$). The MAPK inhibitor U0126 (10µm) significantly reduced LPC induced PLD activation from 860%±309% to 210%±56% (control=100%) (n=6, p=0.006) whilst the TK inhibitors genistein and erbstatin had a partial inhibitory effect. These results indicate that MAPK and tyrosine kinases are involved in LPC induced PLD activation in HUVECs.

PEF 1

PAR-2 ACTIVATION INDUCES JOINT HYPERAEMIA

J.C. Lockhart[1], E.B. Kelso[2], L. Dunning[1], W.R. Ferrell[2]
[1]Biological Sciences, University of Paisley, Paisley, PA1 2BE, [2]Centre for Rheumatic Diseases, University of Glasgow, Glasgow, G31 2ER, UK.

There has been recent interest in protease-activated receptor-2 (PAR-2) as a mediator of neurogenic inflammation. However, PAR-2 is rapidly induced in blood vessels following injury indicating it may mediate non-neurogenic inflammatory responses. We have recently reported a key role for this receptor in a murine model of chronic arthritis [Ferrell, Lockhart, Kelso, Dunning et al. J Clin Invest 2003: 111: 35-41]. The present study investigated the vascular effect of PAR-2 activation in the joint of wild-type (control) and PAR-2 'knock-out' mice.

Mice were deeply anaesthetised using $O_2/N_2O/2\%$ halothane, and the joint exposed by removing an ellipse of skin overlying the joint; the joint was kept irrigated with saline throughout the experiment. All procedures were performed in accordance with current UK regulations. Perfusion in the synovial vasculature was measured using a laser Doppler Imager (LDI; Moor Instruments Ltd, Axminster, UK), and the scans analysed using dedicated software. ASKH95, a selective PAR-2 agonist, was applied topically to the joint at 1 or 10 μg doses, and perfusion changes measured via the sequential scanning facility.

ASKH95, but not a control peptide (ASKH115), significantly increased synovial perfusion in the wild-type mice by 60.4 ± 8.9 % ($P < 0.001$; $n = 7$). This hyperaemia was dose-dependent, maximal after 2 minutes, but was absent in the PAR-2 'knock-out' mice.

These findings demonstrate that PAR-2 activation results in pronounced hyperaemia, a cardinal sign of inflammation. Selectivity of the PAR-2 agonist was established using the 'knock-out' animal, given the current lack of PAR-2 antagonists.

[Study funded by Arthritis Research Campain Grant L0559]

PEF 2

ENDOTHELIAL DYSFUNCTION IN RHEUMATOID ARTHRITIS

W.R Ferrell[1], D. Datta[1], N. Sattar[2], R.D. Sturrock1
[1]Centre for Rheumatic Diseases and [2]Department of Pathological Biochemistry, Glasgow Royal Infirmary, Glasgow, G31 2ER, Scotland, United Kingdom.

Rheumatoid arthritis (RA) has an increased risk of coronary heart disease (CHD). CHD and atherosclerosis are closely linked and associated with vascular dysfunction. Cross-sectional studies show that endothelial function is compromised in RA patients. Inflammation, assessed *in vivo* by C-reactive protein (CRP) levels, is thought to be important in the development of CHD in RA. This study investigates whether vascular function improves as inflammation resolves. Eight RA patients (60.5±4.8 years; mean±SEM) with active disease (CRP>20mg/L or ESR> 30mm/h) gave informed consent to participate. Endothelial function was assessed non-invasively pre- and post- treatment (10.9±2.4 days between scans), by measuring the perfusion response to iontophoretic administration of acetylcholine (ACh; endothelium-dependent) and sodium nitroprusside (SNP; endothelium-independent). Perfusion was assessed non-invasively using a laser Doppler imager (Moor Instruments Ltd, UK). Post-treatment scans showed increased response to ACh ($P<0.002$; 2-way ANOVA), indicating improved vascular responsiveness. The SNP response showed a small, but significant rise ($P=0.049$). CRP decreased from 91±29 to 23±5 mg/L after treatment ($P=0.042$). Analysis of % change in CRP against % change in perfusion showed a significant negative trend ($P=0.02$) i.e. higher pre-treatment CRP is associated with lesser improvement in endothelial function after treatment. Vascular dysfunction in RA patients is detectable non-invasively in the skin microvasculature and improves following anti-inflammatory treatment. The ACh response improves proportionally more than SNP, suggesting that endothelial function is more impaired than vascular smooth muscle during acute 'flare-ups'.

PEF 3

DECREASED CONNEXIN 40 EXPRESSION IN MOUSE RESISTANCE ARTERIES DURING LIPOPOLYSACCHARIDE-INDUCED INFLAMMATION

Y. Ouellette[1], G. Sieck[2]
Department of Pediatrics[1], Physiology & Biomedical Engineering[2], Mayo Clinic College of Medicine, Rochester, MN 55905, USA.

While the effect of sepsis on vascular communication is not well understood, it is known that lipopolysaccharide (LPS) reduces endothelial cell gap junctional intercellular communication in vitro and reduces conducted arteriolar response in vivo. However, changes in the in vivo expression of vascular connexins (gap junction proteins) in response to LPS has not been fully investigated.

In this study, we used immunostaining and RT-PCR to assess connexin content and expression in small mesenteric resistance arteries (diameter ~200 μm) isolated from mice treated with or without intra-peritoneal LPS (5 mg/kg for 6 h). Indirect immunofluorescence on frozen sections of mesenteric resistance arteries demonstrated that connexin 40 (Cx40) and Cx37 were mainly expressed in the endothelial layer, and that Cx43 was found only in some vessels. Connexins were not seen in the media. LPS did not alter distribution of connexins. RT-PCR analysis of Cx expression indicated that LPS treatment caused a reduction in endothelial Cx40 levels. Cx37 levels decreased only slightly after LPS treatment. We detected only small amounts of Cx43 mRNA that remained unchanged after LPS treatment. β-Actin expression (internal control) was not affected by LPS. LPS injection caused a reduction in Cx40 levels in $Cx37^{-/-}$ endothelium, whereas LPS actually decreased Cx37 levels in $Cx40^{-/-}$ endothelium.

These results suggest that LPS mediates changes in endothelial gap junction-mediated communication, at least in part, through modulation of Cx40 and Cx37 levels.

PEF 4

CONTROL OF CA^{2+} SIGNALLING AND MEMBRANE POTENTIAL IN ENDOTHELIAL CELLS OF THE RAT MESENTERIC ARTERY

M.M. Spitaler, C.J. Garland, K.A. Dora
Department of Pharmacy and Pharmacology, University of Bath, Bath, BA2 7AY, UK

In rat mesenteric arteries, ACh increases endothelial cell (EC) intracellular Ca2+ concentration ($[Ca^{2+}]_i$) causing membrane hyperpolariz-ation (HP) through activation of Ca^{2+}-activated K^+ channels (K_{Ca}). In intact arteries, EDHF-mediated relaxation evoked by ACh is abolished by a combination of inhibitors for intermediate- and small-conductance K_{Ca} (IK_{Ca}, SK_{Ca}). In the absence of any tone, smooth muscle HP to ACh is abolished by apamin alone (Crane G et al. J. Physiol 2003; 553.1: 183-189). To investigate the role of endothelial cell ion channels in these responses, ACh-stimulated changes in $[Ca^{2+}]_i$ and membrane potential were measured in freshly isolated sheets of ECs in the presence of the IK_{Ca} and SK_{Ca} inhibitors, TRAM-34 and apamin, respectively.

Membrane potential recordings were obtained using the perforated-patch-clamp technique. Changes in $[Ca^{2+}]_i$ were monitored by loading the cells with fluo-4/AM. In sheets of ECs, ACh stimulated a reproducible HP (DEm=37±5mV, n=3). Apamin alone fully blocked the HP, and ACh stimulated depolarization. ACh also stimulated a rise in Ca^{2+} in isolated sheets of ECs (F/F_0: Peak: 2.48±0.44; 2min: 1.45±0.11; n=5), which was not altered in the presence of apamin (50nM) and TRAM-34 (1μM) (F/F_0: Peak: 1.79±0.14; 2min: 1.27±0.10; n=5). The observation that membrane HP did not drive EC Ca2+ influx was supported by the absence of any change in $[Ca^{2+}]_i$ with high K^+ (35mM) in unstimulated cells.

These data show that in isolated ECs of the mesenteric artery, ACh-mediated HP is evoked by activation of SK_{Ca}, but the driving force for Ca^{2+} influx is unaltered by up to 40mV change in membrane potential. Supported by the Wellcome Trust, UK.

PEF 5

SPECIFICITY AND VIABILITY OF A PINOCYTOTIC METHOD FOR LOADING ENDOTHELIAL CELLS IN INTACT ARTERIES

P. Winter, S.L. Sandow, S. Mather, C.J. Garland, K.A. Dora
Department of Pharmacy and Pharmacology, University of Bath, Bath BA2 7AY, UK.

The ability to pinocytotically load cell impermeant molecules specifically into endothelial cells of intact arteries (Mather et al. J. Physiol 2004; 555P: C10) was verified at the ultrastructural level.
Male Wistar rats (200-250g) were killed humanely (Animals Scientific Procedure Act 1986, UK). Third-order branches of the superior mesenteric artery were isolated, cannulated and pressurised to 50mmHg at 37°C. Following assessment of endothelial cell viability with ACh, the lumen was perfused with hypertonic solution containing 3% myoglobin (17.6kDa) or $5x10^{11}$ 10nm gold-conjugated IgG (150kDa) particles, followed by hypotonic solution and then physiological solution. Vessels were fixed at each stage for electron microscopy using conventional methods.
Endothelial cells in arteries exposed to the loading protocol/hypertonic solution showed a marked increase (approx 10-fold) in 50-100nm diameter spherical cytoplasmic vesicles, and contained a higher density of myoglobin and gold-conjugated IgG than control vessels. The ultrastructural integrity of the endothelium was unaffected by these treatments, and there were no myoglobin or gold-conjugated IgG particles observed outside the intimal layer.
This pinocytotic loading protocol can be used to selectively load large molecular weight cell-membrane impermeable molecules into the endothelium of intact arteries without disrupting vessel integrity. The method will thus enable the functional targeting of endothelial signalling pathways to further elucidate mechanisms involved in the regulation of arterial tone. Supported by the BHF and Wellcome Trust.

PEF 6

VASCULAR DYSFUNCTION AND MARKERS OF ENDOTHELIAL DAMAGE IN HYPERTENSIVE PATIENTS WITH AND WITHOUT END STAGE RENAL DISEASE

K Farkas[1], J Nemcsik[1], E Kolossváry[1], Z Járai[2], J Borvendég[1], Cs Farsang[2], I Kiss[1]
[1]1st Dept. of Int. Med., St. Imre Teaching Hosp., Budapest, Tétényi u. 12-16., 1115-Hungary, [2]1st Dept. of Int. Med, Semmelweis Univ. Budapest

In patients with chronic renal failure and hypertension, the risk for cardiovascular complications is increased. The aim of the study was to evaluate microvascular reactivity in hypertensive patients with and without end stage renal disease using laser Doppler flowmetry. In 34 hypertensive patients (EHT), 21 hypertensive hemodialyzed patients (DHT) and also in 22 normotensive control subjects (CONT) the postocclusive reactive hyperemia test (PORH) and acetylcholine (ACh) and sodium nitroprusside (SNP) iontophoresis were performed on the forearm skin. We measured the serum level of differrent markers as well. The average peakflow for the PORH were 284 ± 26 % (mean ± SEM) in the EHT, 234 ± 48 % in the DHT and 434 ± 36 % in the CONT (p<0,05). The average hyperaemic response to the higher dose of ACh iontophoresis were 531 ± 47 % in EHT, 360 ± 67 % in DHT and 836 ± 97 % in CONT (p<0,05, p<0,001 comp. to CONT). The vasodilation after the higher dose of SNP was 660 ± 72 % in EHT, 379 ± 63 % in DHT and 791 ± 79 % in CONT (NS, p<0,001). Levels of ET-1 and big-ET were over the normal range in EHT (0,80 ± 2.04; 1,29 ± 1.2 fmol/ml) and DHT (1.40 ± 2.87; 2.67 ± 1.61 fmol/l), big-ET was significantly higher (p<0,001) in DHT compared to EHT. vWF level was significantly higher in DHT (174.4 ± 89 %) compared to CONT (90.57 ±16 %, p<0,001). In hypertensive dialyzed patients both the endothelium-dependent and the endothelium-independent vasodilation are impaired and markers of endothelial damage are increased, which may indicate the progress of vascular disease.

PEF 7

EFFECT OF L-NMMA ON SKIN LASER DOPPLER FLUX DURING LOCAL COOLING AND ALPHA-ADRENOCEPTOR AGONISTS ACTION

Strucl M, Cankar K
Institute of Physiology, Medical faculty, Ljubljana, Slovenia

It has been suggested that endothelium derived nitric oxide and alpha 2-adrenoceptor mechanism might interfere at the level of microcirculation in some experimental and pathological conditions. We studied first the effect of intradermal microinjection of synthase inhibitor (L-NMMA) on skin Laser-Doppler (LD) flux at normal skin temperature (34°C), second during local cooling (15°C) and third during the action of alpha 1-agonist (phenylephrin) and alpha 2-agonist (clonidine). LD flux was monitored in the fingertips of 9 healthy volunteers. The study has ethical approval and the patient consent has been obtained from each subject. To evaluate the possible effect of micro trauma we compared the results with those obtained after intradermal microinjection of saline solution. The application of L-NMMA did not cause any significant change of LD-flux at normal temperature and during the cooling. In contrast, L-NMMA significantly reduced LD flux during the action of clonidine from 54 ± 6 PU to 41 ± 6 PU but not during the action of phenylephrine at normal skin temperature (ANOVA, p<0.05). Our results are consistent with the animal preparations studies that endothelium-derived NO mechanism and alpha 2 response interfere in certain conditions. We were able to prove this interference at the level of skin microcirculation in the condition of maximum alpha 2 agonist activation.

PEF 8

THE EFFECT OF A EVENING HIGH FAT MEAL ON ENDOTHELIAL FUNCTION IN YOUNG WOMEN

S.M.Hampton, G.Salkeld, L.James, J.F.Walters,G.A AFerns[1] and D.J.Skene
Neuroendocrinology Group, [1]Centre for Clinical Science and Measurement, School of Biomedical and Molecular Sciences, University of Surrey, Guildford, Surrey, GU21 7XH, UK

This study investigated the effect of a late evening high fat meal on endothelial function in young women. Ethical Committee approval was obtained. Seven women, aged (22 ± 0.8 years [mean ± SD]), and all on a combined oral contraceptive pill were studied on two occasions following high and low fat meals. Subjects remained awake and sedentary in dim light conditions (<5lux) throughout the study. Subjects were either given a high fat meal (47% fat, 35% carbohydrate, 18% protein) or a low fat meal (15% fat, 64% carbohydrate, 31% protein) at 2000 h. Endothelium-dependent flow mediated dilatation (FMD) was assessed by high-resolution ultrasound of the branchial artery prior to the meal, and 2 and 4 h post meal. Baseline and hourly blood samples were taken. Two way repeated measure ANOVA showed no significant difference in %FMD between the two meals however a significant difference was observed over time (P=0.05). The lowest %FMD occured prior to the meals and the greatest responses was observed 6h postprandially. Significant differences were observed in plasma post-prandial triacylglycerol levels (TAG) after both fat meals (*P*= 0.007). Peak TAG levels occurred 4h after the high fat meal with low fat meal TAG responses remained low thoughout the study. These preliminary results show that a meal consumed at night did not impair endothelial function at 2 and 6 h post meal. Since peak TAG levels occurred 4 h after the high fat meal, future studies will need to assess endothelial function at that time.

PEF 9

CIRCADIAN RHYTHM IN CARDIOVASCULAR FUNCTION IN WOMEN UNDER CONSTANT ROUTINE CONDITIONS

J.F Walters[1], S.M Hampton[1], J.E Deanfield[3], A.E Donald[3], D.J Skene1 and G.A.A Ferns[2]
[1]Neuroendocrinology Group, [2]Centre for Clinical Science and Measurement, School of Biomedical and Molecular Sciences, University of Surrey, Guildford, Surrey, GU2 7XH, UK, [3]Vascular Physiology Dept, Great Ormond Street Hospital for Children, London, UK

The present study was undertaken to investigate the existence of endogenously generated circadian rhythms in endothelial function, blood pressure and heart rate in women and whether the rhythm is altered after the menopause. Ethical approval was obtained from the University of Surrey Ethics Committee. Eleven healthy pre-menopausal (n = 11) and postmenopausal (n = 10) women were studied, during a 22 h period under conditions of constant dim light (< 10 lux), temperature, posture, meal intake and maintained wakefulness. Flow-mediated dilatation (%FMD) and glyceryl trinitrate (GTN)-mediated dilatation was assessed by high-resolution ultrasound of the brachial artery. Blood pressure and heart rate was also determined hourly. A significant day-night variation in %FMD was observed in pre-menopausal women (day 9.1 ± 0.8; night 10.2 ± 1; mean ± SEM) ($P < 0.05$). This rhythm was attenuated in postmenopausal women (day 6.8 ± 0.6; night 6.0 ± 0.4). No variation over time was observed in GTN-mediated dilatation in either study group. A circadian rhythm in both systolic and diastolic blood pressure and heart rate was also observed in both pre-menopausal and postmenopausal women. Systolic blood pressure was significantly increased ($P < 0.05$) in postmenopausal women. The findings show evidence of an endogenous circadian rhythm in endothelium-dependent function (% FMD) in pre-menopausal women, which is attenuated after the menopause.

PEF 10

MYOENDOTHELIAL COUPLING IS NOT PROMINENT IN MURINE ARTERIOLES IN VIVO

C. de Wit*, D. Siegl#, KBM. Koeppen#, U. Pohl#
*Physiologisches Institut, Universität Lübeck, Ratzeburger Allee 160, 23538 Lübeck, Germany; #Physiolog. Institut, LMU, München, Germany

The membrane potential (MP) is an important determinant of microvascu-lar tone. The endothelium contributes to the control of smooth muscle MP by EDHF and/or direct current transfer via gap junctions. MP was measured in vascular cells with microelectrodes in vivo during acetylcholine (ACh) stimulation in the cremaster of mice. Endothelial cell (EC) or vascular smooth muscle (VSM) were identified according to their orientation to the vessel after staining via the measuring pipette.

MP at rest was lower in EC than in VSM (-47.6±0.5 vs. –37.1±0.9 mV). Locally confined stimulation with ACh induced robust hyperpolarisations (HYP) in EC and VSM, which were, however, significantly larger in EC than in VSM. In the presence of charybdotoxin (blocker of BKCa) HYP upon ACh were abrogated in VSM (from -4.3±1.4 mV to +1.0±1.3 mV, n=7), but MP changes in EC remained unaffected (-10.3±1.1 vs. -9.9±0.6 mV, n=7). Similar results were obtained with the more specific blocker iberiotoxin. In contrast, apamin, a blocker of SKCa-channels, attenuated HYP in EC upon ACh significantly (from -6.7±1.1 to -2.0± 1.1 mV, n=6) and had only a minor effect in VSM (from -5.5±2.3 to -3.3± 1.2mV, n=6). Dilations upon ACh (3μM) were attenuated by iberiotoxin from 50±5 to 13 ±4%, while apamin reduced the responses only from from 53±4 to 31±5%.

These data demonstrate that myoendothelial coupling is not the major determinant of MP in vascular cells. EC and VSM differ with respect to resting MP, response upon ACh, and type of Ca^{2+}-dependent K^+-channel mediating the hyperpolarisation upon ACh, i.e. BKCa in VSM and predominantly SKCa in EC. The mechanical dilation is mainly dependent on the activation of BKCa.

PEF 11

RHEUMATOID ARTHRITIS ALTERS CAPILLARY RECRUITMENT IN THE SKIN

D.A. Warland, R.C. Haigh, M. Beaman, A.C.Shore
Clinical Microvascular Research Unit, ICBS, Peninsula Medical School, Barrack Road, Exeter, EX2 5AX, UK

Rheumatoid arthritis is associated with conduit vessel endothelial dysfunction. We examined whether rheumatoid arthritis is associated with microvascular dysfunction.

14 patients with rheumatoid arthritis (RA) were compared with 14 healthy subjects. The local research ethics committee approved the study and all patients gave written informed consent. Capillary density was assessed in the resting state and after 10 minutes of venous occlusion in the skin of the dorsal middle finger, middle phalanx to determine capillary maximal density. In addition capillaries perfused continuously over a 15 s period were counted at rest and immediately after 4 minutes of arterial occlusion – this was performed on the index finger 1.5mm proximal to the terminal row of capillaries in the nailbed.

There was no significant difference in capillary density at rest, after venous occlusion or after arterial occlusion. The percentage increase in capillary number after venous occlusion was greater in the RA group vs healthy group (10.4 vs 6.1% p<0.05). Continuously perfused capillary recruitment after arterial occlusion (that is the increase in number divided by baseline number x 100) was less in the RA group vs healthy group (76 vs 112% p<0.05).

The results suggest capillary density is not altered in rheumatoid arthritis but the pattern of capillary perfusion is. In patients with rheumatoid arthritis the proportion of capillaries perfused at rest is lower but they are perfused for a greater proportion of time. Rheumatoid arthritis has an effect on microcircula-tory function as well as large vessel function.

PEF 12

PREDICTORS OF SKIN MINIMUM VASCULAR RESISTANCE IN HEALTHY SUBJECTS

K.M.Gooding, J.L.Whatmore, D.Warland, M.M.Hannemann, A.R.Middlebrooke, K.Paisley, W.Liddell, B.Lee, J.E.Tooke, A.C.Shore
Institute of Biomedical and Clinical Science, Peninsula Medical School, Barrack Road, Exeter, EX2 5AX, UK

Skin maximum hyperaemia to local heating was assessed in healthy Caucasian subjects (n= 117; 49 males; age range: 20-86yrs). Minimum vascular resistance (MVR) was calculated to normalise for variations in blood pressure (mean arterial pressure/max. hyperaemia). Blood samples were assayed for cholesterol, triglycerides, fasting insulin and glucose. Insulin sensitivity was calculated with fasting insulin and glucose using HOMA. In univariate analysis, MVR was negatively associated with insulin sensitivity (r= -0.220, p= 0.021, Pearson). To examine this relationship further multiple regression was performed with insulin resistance markers: age, body mass index (BMI), cholesterol and triglycerides. Sub group analysis based on gender and menopausal status was then performed to examine their impact on the relationship between insulin senstivity and MVR. Cholesterol and BMI were significant predictors of MVR in all subjects (R square:0.112,0.05 respectively, F-ratio:10.981, p<0.001). Sub group analysis based on gender revealed that triglycerides were predictors of MVR in men (R square: 0.162, F-ratio: 9.112, p= 0.004) while cholesterol and BMI were predictors of MVR in women (R square: 0.132,0.059, F-ratio: 8.717, p<0.001). Subgroup analysis based on menopausal status revealed that cholesterol was a predictor of MVR in premenopausal women (R square: 0.238, F-ratio: 14.024, p= 0.001). In postmenopausal women, age was a predictor of MVR (R square: 0.161, F-ratio: 5.169, p= 0.031). Thus in healthy subjects insulin sensitivity is negatively related to MVR, but the factors contributing to this relationship vary with gender and menopausal status.

PEF 13

SPECTRAL ANALYSIS OF BLOOD FLUX OSCILLATIONS IN HUMAN SKIN – A TOOL FOR ASSESSING RISK

M.R. Avery, G.F.Clough
Infection, Inflammation and Repair, School of Medicine, University of Southampton, Southampton, SO16 6YD, UK.

Analysis of the oscillations in skin blood flux recorded using the non- invasive technique of laser Doppler fluximetry reveals five characteristic frequencies: cardiac and respiratory rhythms (1 and 0.3 Hz) and three others around 0.1, 0.04 and 0.01 Hz. These are thought to reflect myogenic neurogenic and endothelium-mediated activity of the peripheral vasculature, respectively (Kvandel et al Microvasc Res 2003;65:160-171).

We hypothesise that an altered local vascular perfusion may be an early indicator of risk for skin breakdown. To investigate this we explored whether alterations in local oscillations could be detected in a group of moderate to heavy smokers. Cutaneous blood flux was measured using laser Doppler fluximetry (LDF) (Moor Instruments UK) before, during and after 10 minutes local heating to 43°C, in 10 smokers (range 12.5 - 42 pack years) and healthy controls matched for age, sex and BMI. The shape of the response to thermal heating was similar in both smokers and non-smokers. However, analysis of the LDF signal in the time domain, showed that the smokers had a 31 ± 11.4 % reduction in peak flux, with the total vasodilatory response to heating being attenuated by 34.2 ± 24.3 % (mean ± sem) ($P<0.01$). Evaluation of the LDF signal in the frequency domain between 0.008 and 2.0 Hz, using Fourier transformation, showed oscillations at the frequency interval 0.008-0.02 Hz and 0.09 – 0.11 Hz to be significantly attenuated in the smokers compared with non-smokers, during both the baseline flux and plateau response to heating ($P<0.05$).

The results suggest that smoking results in early and detectable changes in the regulation of cutaneous vascular perfusion and that these are a result of changes in vascular endothelial and smooth muscle cell activity.

PEF 14

LOW POTASSIUM DEXTRANE PRESERVES CRITICAL ENDOTHELIAL FUNCTION DURING TEMPORARY STORAGE OF VENOUS GRAFTS IN CORONARY BYPASS SURGERY.

Eifert S[1], Kronschnabl M[1], Vicol C[1], Chouker A[2], Reichart B[1] and Christ F[2].
Depts. of Cardiac Surgery[1] and Anesthesiology[2], Ludwig Maximilians University Munich, Germany

Background:
For several years Perfadex, a low-potassium dextrane solution (LPD), has been used to preserve endothelial function during organ storage for lung transplantation. As the integrity of bypass graft endothelium seems to be essential for successful long-term patency in coronary bypass surgery, its preservation demands the utmost care. The aim of the present study was to investigate the effects of currently used solutions (Bretschneider/ fresh heparinized blood) on endothelial function after short-term storage of venous bypass grafts at room temperature and compare it to veins stored in Perfadex.
Methods and Material.
We distinguished two patient's groups: group I (n= 20), received Perfadex for venous graft storage between harvest and anastomosing and group II (n=20), veins were stored in Bretschneider's cardioplegic solution. In all patients blood samples were investigated for myocardial encymes, Interleukin 6 and TNF alpha preoperatively and at the beginning and end of CPB as well as postoperatively (every 6 hours for two days). Leucocyte adhesion markers were examined at same time points by FITS and endothelial function evaluated. Additionally, samples of veins were taken and histology was examined in each patient to investigate destruction of endothelium.
Results.
As Perfadex prevents endothelial damage we obtained the following results: Cytokine measurements and myocardial encyme levels did not show significant differences in both groups. Leucocyte adhesion markers such as IB4 and D200 levels and CD-11b counts respectively, were diminished in group I. The endothelial damage in group I was less than in group II due to Perfadex preservation. Histology did not showa significant difference in both groups..
Conclusions.
Perfadex prevents early endothelial dysfunction as good as Bretschneider cardioplegic solution at room temperature.

PEF 15

THE STUDY OF VELNACRINE MALEATE EFFECTS ON ENDOTHELIAL CELL SECOND MESSENGERS

F.A. Carvalho, C. Saldanha, J. Martins-Silva
Instituto de Bioquímica, Faculdade de Medicina de Lisboa. Unidade de Biopatologia Vascular, IMM, 1649-028 Lisboa, Portugal.

In the endothelial cell signal transduction pathways there are several receptors which have acetylcholine (ACh) as agonist. Acetylcholinesterase that hydrolyses ACh is also present. We studied the effect of ACh on the NO production and on the cAMP and cGMP concentration, on cultured HUVECs, in the absence or in the presence of velnacrine maleate (VM, acetylcholinesterase inhibitor).

Cultured cells were allowed to stabilize for 30 minutes in PBS buffer. After that, we stimulated the HUVECs with ACh 10 μM in absence or in presence of VM 10 μM and monitorized the HUVECs NO production with a amperometric NO sensor. HUVECs stimulated with ACh (0, 0.01μM, 1 μM and 10 μM) in absence or in presence of VM 10 μM, were lysed and assayed for quantification of total cellular cAMP and cGMP.

We observed that ACh induced an increase on NO production and this effect was significantly lowered in presence of VM ($P=0.009$, $n=5$). The cAMP and cGMP levels increased upon incubation with ACh. For ACh 10μM, the cAMP levels were of 16.7 fmol/well vs 4.1 fmol/well (control) and the cGMP levels were of 2.3 fmol/well vs 1.7 fmol/well (control), as an example. The VM slightly reduced those levels. This cAMP decrease was more evident for high ACh concentrations while the cGMP levels decrease was more relevant for low ACh concentrations.

In conclusion, these results revealed that the ACh activate the signal transduction mechanisms that leads to the NO, cAMP and cGMP production in HUVECs. The AChE-VM complex interfere with these mechanisms that so far are unknown.

Friday, 10th September
Poster Presentation – Haemodynamics and Vascular Responses (PHD)

PHD 1

SMALL ARTERIAL ELASTANCE CAN BE USED TO ESTIMATE ENDOTHELIAL FUNCTION

R. Draijer, C.I. Wright, K.A.J. Brouwer, C. Kroner
Unilever Health Institute, Vlaardingen, The Netherlands

Flow-mediated dilation (FMD) is commonly used to assess endothelial function, even though recorded responses can be quite variable. A suggested alternative is pulse wave analysis (PWA) using CR-2000 tonometer (Hypertension Diagnostics Inc.). Presently, however, it is unclear how these two methods correlate and so in the present study we assessed this. 12 (8 males and 4 females) healthy volunteers with a mean age of 35±10 (mean±S.D.) were enrolled in a randomised, crossover designed study. FMD was monitored using echosonography and maximally induced increases in arterial diameter (% changes) were recorded using the Walltrack® system (PieMedical). FMD brachial arterial responses were determined in the forearm (by occluding the upperarm) and upperarm (forearm occlusion), where a pressure cuff was inflated to 200 mmHg for a maximum of 5 minutes. These responses were correlated with large (LAE) and small arterial elastance (SAE), which were recorded in resting individuals immediately after the FMD measurements had been conducted. SAE and LAE were determined using PWA of the radial artery. FMD responses tended to be larger in the forearm than the upperarm (5.7±2.6 vs. 4.6±2.6%). Average SAE and LAE were 9.5±3.2 ml mmHg^{-1} x100 and 17.9±4.4 ml mmHg^{-1} x10. SAE significantly correlated with forearm FMD responses (R^2=0.51, *P*=0.01) but not the upperarm (R^2=0.06, *P*>0.05). No relations existed for FMD and LAE. Finally, the intra-subject coefficient of variance for SAE and LAE was 13.0 and 7.7% respectively. Forearm FMD responses correlated well with SAE and so PWA seems a feasible alternative for non-invasively measuring endothelial function. Further support for its use is that it has a low intra-subject coefficient of variance (some 3-4 times less than FMD).

PHD 2

A MODIFIED BROOKSBY-DONALD (B-D) APPROACH TO MEASURE TRANSIENT SYSTEMIC CONDUCTANCE AND CAPACITANCE RESPONSES IN ANESTHETISED RABBITS.

Wright CI, Roach D, Thakore E, Sheldon RS, Tyberg JV.
Cardiovascular Research Group, University of Calgary, Alberta, Canada.

Originally, the B-D method was developed to measure venous capacitance and did so by time-integrating the difference between sub-diaphragmatic inflow and outflow. We modified this method to measure transient responses of both venous capacitance and arterial conductance (1/vascular resistance) and demonstrate its usefulness by showing transient vasodilator (to nitroglycerin, NG) and constrictor (phenylephrine, PE) responses. In fentanyl-anaesthetised (1.6-4.2mg kg^{-1} min^{-1} iv), artificially ventilated rabbits, ultrasonic flow probes were affixed to the descending thoracic aorta and inferior vena cava at the level of the diaphragm and changes in capacitance were estimated by time-integrating their difference. Changes in arterial conductance were calculated by dividing aortic flow by the difference between sub-diaphragmatic arterial and venous pressures. PE, given in a 2-fold step-wise manner (0.5-8 μg kg^{-1}; n=8), maximally decreased capacitance and conductance by 0.36±0.18 ml kg^{-1} and 39.5±6.8% (mean±SEM), respectively, with conductance decreasing at each dose and capacitance only changing at the highest dose tested. NG, given in a similar fashion (range, 1-16μg kg^{-1}; n=8), maximally increased capacitance and conductance by 0.31±0.10 ml kg^{-1} and 155.8±9.39% at doses of 4 and 16 mg kg^{-1} respectively. However, whilst NG increased conductance at each dose, near maximal changes in capcitance were reached at the lowest dose. We have demonstrated the usefulness of this modified B-D approach by showing both dilatory responses to NG and constrictor responses to PE. This method would be of use for defining the cardiovascular effects of various vasoactive agents.

PHD 3

WAVELENGTH AND PROBE CONFIGURATION OF LASER DOPPLER DEVICES

C. Freccero, P. Wollmer*, G. Sundkvist**, H. Svensson
From the Departments of Plastic and Reconstructive Surgery, *Clinical Physiology and **Endocrinology, Malmo University Hospital, University of Lund, SE-20502 Malmo, Sweden.

The aim of the present study was to investigate to what degree a standardised test for assessing sympathetic skin vasoconstriction based on laser Doppler blood flow measurement is dependent on the particular equipment set-up being used. As a part of our programme for development of clinical devices and procedures, we therefore examined 20 healthy subjects with a median age of 47 years.

Laser Doppler Perfusion Monitoring (LDPM) with fibre separations 0.25 and 1.2 mm, and Laser Doppler Perfusion Imaging (LDPI) with 633 and 780 nm wavelengths were used. The hand was placed in a supporting holder with a temperature of 40°C. Contra-lateral cooling was achieved by immersing hand and forearm in water of 15°C. To obtain a numerical expression of the decrease in blood flow, the lowest perfusion value during the first minute of cooling was divided by the mean value of two minutes before cooling. We thus constructed a vasoconstriction index (VAC).

VAC values (mean) were 0.556 for LDPM-0.25, 0.561 for LDPM-1.2, 0.668 for LDPI-633, and 0.629 for LDPI-780. VAC for LDPI-633 differed significantly (p=0.012) from the others.

Presumably due to different volumes being probed with different distances between illuminating and receiving fibres in LDPM, and different wavelengths in LDPI, responses may vary also when using a standardised test like ours. Although differences were found to be minor, this fact must be considered for instance when comparing results from one laboratory to another.

PHD 4

ACTIVE DILATATION OF VENULAR MICROVESSELS DURING MODERATE ARTERIAL HYPOTENSION

1. Tatarishvili, T .Sordia, G.Mchedlishvili Microcirculation Research Center, IBeritashvili Institute ofPhysiology, 14 Gotua S1., 0160 Tbilisi, Georgia.

Since the middle of the 20 th century it became generally accepted that the microvascular network vasomotor activity is characteristic only for the smallest arterioles and initial parts of the thoroughfare channels, possessing muscular elements in their walls. As to the other parts of the network, it were believed to be deprived not only fo any contractive elements in their walls, but also of any kind of vasomotor activity.
In experiments on white laboratory rats intestinal mesenterium, using the Leitz Wentslar intravital videomicroscopical technique we assessed the microvascular diameters of the identified arteriolar and venular parts of the throughfare channels. The obtained results were treated statistically by using of Student's paired T test.
We found that during controled lowering of systemic arterial pressure (caused by hemorrhage) up to 50 per cent, the arteriolar microvessels contracted, while the diameters of capillary venular portions (15-30 J.lm wide) increased by a mean of 26 per cent, respectively.
We conjecture that the venular dilatation might be a compensatory response directed to maintenance of blood flow in the capillary network, but in 18 nature and physiological mechanisms remain the unclear, unlike the arterial constriction, which is directed to maintain the systemic arterial pressure.

PHD 5

THE EFFECT OF DIAZEPAM ON GENDER DIFFERENCES IN CUTANEOUS LD FLUX RESPONSE TO LOCAL COOLING

Z Melik, K Cankar
Institute of Physiology, Medical faculty, Ljubljana, Slovenia

Several investigators have observed sex differences in cutaneous vascular response to local cooling. The response is greater in females. It is known that cold induces amplification of alpha2 adrenoceptor affinity for noradrenaline and increases reflex sympathetic thermoregulatory output. The difference in the response to cold between males and females could be result of either of both mechanisms. Benzodiazepines in high doses used in clinical practise influence arterial blood pressure, peripheral resistance and heart rate. Moreover, they also act synergistically with alpha adrenoceptor agonists. Both effects could be observed in the response of cutaneous microcirculation to cold. To distinguish between both components; we studied the effect of orally applied diazepam (5mg) on cutaneous microcirculatory response to local cooling at the site of cold exposure. Laser-Doppler (LD) flux was measured in the group of 9 males and 11 females (before and during local cooling of hand at 15°C) in the fingertips (direct response). The study has ethical approval and the patient consent has been obtained from each subject. We also monitored the arterial blood pressure and the heart rate. The obtained values before and one hour after application of diazepam were compared by paired t-test. Our results show that diazepam in low dose augments the direct LD flux response to cold in the group of females. The relative LD flux value changed from 62,5 ± 8% to 49,6 ± 5% ($p<0,05$). In the group of males LD flux did not change. The sympathetic tone did not change after the diazepam application. It seems possible that the greater response to cold in females is the result of the interaction between diazepam and alpha2 adrenoceptors. The alpha2 adrenoceptors are known to have a greater role in females than in males.

PHD 6

THE EFFECT OF CALCIUM-BLOCKERS ON CUTANEOUS POSTOCCLUSIVE REACTIVE HYPERAEMIA

Cankar K, Strucl M
Institute of Physiology, Medical faculty, Ljubljana, Slovenia

L-type and T-type Ca^{2+} channels have been demonstrated to control the activity of the vascular smooth muscles. It is not clear which Ca^{2+} channel type plays predominant role at the level of microcirculation in humans. We aimed to clarify the role of L-type and T-type Ca^{2+} channels at the level of skin microcirculation. For this purpose we studied the effect of distinct Ca^{2+} channel blockers on the skin postocclusive reactive hyperaemia (PRH). The laser-Doppler (LD) flux was monitored in 10 healthy volunteers at the skin of the fingertips before and after an 8-minute occlusion of the digital arteries. The study has ethical approval and the patient consent has been obtained from each subject. The measurements were repeated after an intradermal microinjection of L-type Ca^{2+} channel blocker diltiazem and nimodipine which in addition to L-type Ca^{2+} channels suppresses also T-type Ca^{2+} channels, at the measuring site. The effect of the saline solution injection was used as a reference value. The injection of diltiazem or nimodipine significantly increased resting LD flux values from 267 ± 29 PU to 355 ± 29 or 348 ± 42 PU respectively (ANOVA, $p<0.05$). In contrast, only the application of nimodipine significantly increased the time in which LD flux during the PRH response decreases to the half of its peak LD flux value (T/2) from 20 ± 3 s to 28 ± 4 s, while diltiazem did not affect T/2 of the PRH. Neither of both Ca^{2+} channel blockers influenced the peak LD flux during PRH. Our finding supports the hypothesis about the predominant role of the T-type Ca^{2+} channel in the cutaneous PRH.

PHD 7

CEREBRAL BLOOD FLOW REGULATION IN ANESTHETIZED MORPHINE DEPENDENT RAT

Sohrab Hajizadeh,M.Zahedi, S.Semnanian, Y. Fathollahi
Dept. of physiology, School of Med. Sci.,Tarbiat modarres university P.O.Box 14115-111,Tehran-I.R. Iran

Cerebral cortical blood flow responses to adenosine receptors agonists and antagonists were studied in morphine-naive and dependent rats, using Laser-Doppler flowmetry technique. Adult male Sprague Dawley rats were used in all experiments. Animals were made morphine dependent by administration of morphine sulfate and 3% sucrose in drinking water for 21 days. Results obtained in this study showed that Adenosine (10^{-5}, 10^{-4}, 10^{-3}M) increased regional cerebral blood flow (rCBF) of control, sham-operated and morphine-dependent rat (MDR) in a dose dependent manner, but the amount of increase in MDR was significantly ($P<0.01$) higher than that in control and sham-operated groups. This response was inhibited by theophylline (5_10^{-5}M). N6-cyclohexyladenosine (10^{-6}, 10^{-5}, 10^{-4} M) and 8-cyclopentyltheophylline (10^{-6}M) as selective agonist and antagonist of adenosine A_1-receptor had no effect on rCBF in control, sham-operated and morphine-dependent groups. The enhancing effect of adenosine A_{2a}-receptor agonist (CGS-21680,10^{-6}M) in MDR was abolished by ZM-241385, 10^{-6}M. Adenosine A_{2b}-receptor agonist, 5'-N-ethylcarboxamido-adenosine (NECA, 10^{-6}M) also increased rCBF in MDR. This effect was antagonized by alloxazine, (benzo[g] pteridine-2,4(1H,3H) -dione). Based on these results it is concluded that the vasodilative effect of adenosine or its receptor agonists is augmented in MDR and the greater vasodilation evoked in MDR indicates an increased responsiveness of adenosine A_2 receptors.

PHD 8

INWARD REMODELING OF RESISTANCE ARTERIES: STUCK IN BIOLOGICAL GLUE

E.N.T.P. Bakker[1]; C.L. Buus[2]; J. Perree[1]; A. Ganga[1]; O. Sorop[1], J.A.E. Spaan[1]; T. Rolf[1], M.J. Mulvany[2] and E. VanBavel[1].
[1]Department of Medical Physics, Cardiovascular Research Institute Amsterdam, Academic Medical Center, Amsterdam, the Netherlands
[2]Department of Pharmacology, University of Aarhus, Aarhus, Denmark

Vascular remodeling results in a change in arterial diameter under fully dilated conditions. We hypothesized that inward remodeling is determined by the cross-linking of extracellular matrix proteins by tissue-type transglutaminase (tTG). In vivo, ligation of mesenteric arteries resulted in inward remodeling in 2 days of 18 +/- 3% at 60 mmHg. Injections with tTG inhibitor cystamine reduced the inward remodeling to 9 +/- 3% (n=4). Small porcine coronary arteries (200 microns) were maintained in organoid culture for 3 days at 60 mmHg. These arteries expressed tTG. Comparison of the maximal diameter on day 0 to day 3 showed inward remodeling, of 9 +/- 3% at 60 mmHg (n=7). Upregulation of tTG with retinoic acid (10^{-7} M) resulted in increased vasoconstriction and doubled inward remodeling: 18 +/- 4% (n=6). Inhibition of tTG during culture with cadaverine induced vasodilation and reversed remodeling to: +26 +/- 5% (n=5). Exogenous transglutaminase induced inward remodeling in 24 hours: -10 +/- 3% (n=9) vs. +2 +/- 1% in control arteries (n=7). The effect was completely inhibited by simultaneous addition of the nitric oxide donor nitroprusside (0.1 mM): +4 +/- 2% (n=6). A collagen gel contraction assay showed that TG increased contraction from 64 +/- 3% to only 23 +/- 3% of the original diameter. Inhibition of tTG reduced compaction, to 89 +/- 2%. In conclusion, these data reveal a novel mechanism of vascular remodeling, based on tissue-type transglutaminase.
Supported by the Netherlands Heart Foundation (2001D038 and 98.180).

PHD 9

MICROVASCULAR CORRELATES OF EARLY RENAL DISEASE

[1]A.C Shore, [2]N. Chaturvedi, [2]C.J.Bulpitt, [2]C. Rajkumar, [2]W.D Strain.
[1]Peninsula Medical School, Exeter, United Kingdom, [2]Imperial College School of Medicine, London, United Kingdom.

Background: Hypertension and diabetes are commonly associated with renal damage, thought to be driven by microcirculatory disturbances although the exact mechanisms are unclear. Study of the skin microcirculation using laser Doppler fluximetry provides a non-invasive assessment of such disturbances.
Methods: Time to peak hyperaemic response after a 3-minute arterial occlusion was assessed on a population sample of 47 white Europeans with diabetes and 108 without, aged 40-64. Albumin excretion rate (AER) and albumin creatinine ratio (ACR) were calculated from a timed overnight urine collection.
Results: Two patterns of peak response were observed; a slow rise to a peak at an average of 10.5 seconds (25th, 75th percentiles; 7.6, 15.8s) and a rapid rise to peak in under 1.5 seconds (mean 0.8s (0.8, 1.2s)). Rapid responders had a higher AER (10.8 (4.0, 22.8) vs. 4.4 (2.9, 6.0)μg/min; $p=0.002$). This could not be accounted for by age, height, weight, BP, diabetes status, fasting triglycerides or fasting insulin (b regression coefficient of AER vs. time 0.761±0.306; $p=0.015$). ACR showed a similar association (adjusted β 0.865±0.239; $p<0.001$). Diabetics were 2.3 times more likely to respond rapidly (95% CI 1.1-4.9; $p=0.044$) and BP was positively associated with a rapid peak (b 0.0025±0.0012; $p=0.045$)
Conclusions: A rapid peak hyperaemic response following an ischaemic stimulus is associated with an elevated AER and ACR, and is associated with diabetes. This may represent a failure of autoregulation at the arteriolar level, which could result in transmission of fluctuations in blood pressure to the glomerular capillary bed.

PHD 10

A NON-INVASIVE OPTICAL TECHNIQUE FOR MONITORING CHANGES IN MUSCLE BLOOD FLOW

L-G. Lindberg, M. Sandberg
Department of Biomedical Engineering, 581 85 Linköping, Sweden

In Photoplethysmography(PPG) light from a light source, e.g. a LED, is directed toward the skin and this light is absorbed and scattered in the tissue. A small amount of this light is received by a photodetector placed e.g. adjacent to the LED (reflection mode). Variations in the photodetector signal is related to changes in blood flow and blood volume in the underlying tissue. The light penetration depth depends on the optical wavelength and the distance between the light source and the photodetector.
Assessment of blood flow changes to various provocations, such as post-exercise hyperemia and hyperemia following the application of liniment. Simultaneous measurements using ultrasound Doppler and the new PPG application were performed. Changes in both superficial and deep blood flow was measured before and after the interventions.
Following static and dynamic contractions an immediate increase in muscle blood flow was shown, without increase in skin blood flow. Liniment application to the skin induced a rapid increase in skin blood flow, but not in muscle blood flow.
In conclusion the new custom-designed technique enable;
- non-invasive and continous monitoring of changes in muscle blood flow and blood volume
- an increased understanding of the factors involved in both central and local regulation of blood flow in muscles

PHD 11

INTRA-AND EXTRACELLULAR REGULATORY MECHANISMS OF RBC AGGREGATION

A.S.Petrochenko; A.V.Muravyov, V.V.Yakusevich Yaroslavl State Medical Academy, 150000, Russia

The aim: Red blood cell aggregation (RBCA) contributes significantly to postcapillary resistance, which effects transcapillary exchange. RBCs have both types of adre-noreceptors. A possible aggregation regulatory mechanism is adrenergic. Local aggregation changes may have prostaglandins (PG) as their triggers. To test this hypotheses we examined aggregation of RBCs incubated with α and β-agonists: adrenalin *(A)*, noradrenalin (N), phenilephrine(Ph), clonidine (C), isoproterenol (I) and PG: PGF_1, PGE_2, and $PGF_{2\alpha}$). All catecholamines (CA) were used in micromole concentrations (2.3-4.9^{8} M).
Results: The effect of CA is dose-dependent. All of them stimulated RBCA. An α-2-agonist C produced the most significant effect (+ 156%), N - +150%, and A- +98%. β-agonists had a less significant effect on RBCA (+32%). CA could be placed in such sequence according to their RBCA-stimulation ability: C tN A IR. Dibutyryl cAMP (dB-cAMP) reduced RBCA considerably (by 40- 50%). Combination of CA and dD-cAMP reduced significantly an increase in RBCA produced by CA alone. Blocking of Ca^{2+} channels and Ca^{2+}-chelating with EGTA also decreased RBCA (by 35-46%). A+Verapamil combination stimulated RBCA less than adrenaline alone. On the other hand RBC incubation with Ca^{2+} -ionophore A23187 (1.0 M) produced an almost two-fold increase of RBCA. RBC incubation with PGE_2, $PGF_{2\alpha}$, increased RBCA, and PGE_1 decreased RBCA.
Conclusion. The obtained data evidence that CA and prostaglandins affect RBCA considerably and may be viewed as important signalling pathways. Intracellular mechanism of these changes is probably a competitive interaction of two second messengers; adenilate cyclase and Ca^{2+} calmodulin.

Poster Presentation – Haemodynamics and Vascular Responses (PHT)

PHT 1

DETERMINANT OF CD 62P AND CD 63 RECEPTORS AS ACTIVATED PLATELETS MARKERS IN HYPERTENSIVE PATIENTS

C. Homentcovschi, M. Muraru, H. Bumbea, I. Bruckner
Coltea Clinical Hospital, I.C. bratianu 1-3, sect 3, Bucharest, Romania zip code 030171

Objective: In this study we investigated the platelet activation in hypertensive patients (either with or without diabetes mellitus) by studying membrane antigen expression CD 62P (P selection) and CD 63 (marker of activated platelets secretion).
Design and Methods: We studied 50 patients, divided in three groups: Group 1=12 subjects without high blood pressure, group 2=18 patients with hypertension, but no diabetes and group 3=20 patients with both hypertension and diabetes mellitus. The platelets were normal as number and function; using flowcytometry, we measured the population of platelets that exhibit CD 62P, CD 63 and both. The three groups were homogenous regarding age, gender and antihypertensive treatment.
Results: In hypertensive patients, the expression of CD 62P is greater than in non-hypertensive subjects (7.67% in group 2 and 6.6% in group 3, versus 0.43% in group 1). The values for CD 63 are as follows: 0.24% in group 1, 3.37% in group 2 and 1.69% in group 3. Regarding mix activation (CD 62P/ CD 63), the values are: 0.51% in group 1, 8.46% for the group 2 and 5.29% or group 3. All the results are for a P value < 0.01%.
Conclusions: Platelets activation is superior in hypertensive subjects when we compare with non-hypertensive subjects. The membrane activation is almost the same in hypertensive groups (with or without diabetes mellitus). In hypertensive patients without diabetes, contrary to our expectations has a greater platelet secretion activation, comparing with diabetic patients, implying an indeterminate factor.

PHT 2

THROMBOGENESIS IN RAT DEHYDRATION MODEL

Hiroaki Natsui, Lee Hoseong, Takayuki Akimoto, Kennichi Yanagi, Norio Ohshima and Ichiro Kono
Shimazaki Hospital for Orthopedic Surgery, 2-7-15 Bentencho, Hitachi, Ibaraki 317-0072, JAPAN

Object: Dehydration is serious problem in sport medicine, which occur negative in/out balance of fluid. Dehydration induces such as heat stroke, wight control disturbance or long-flight thrombosis. It is important to evaluate thrombogenesis in microcirculatory level. We intended to observe thrombogenesis using intra-vital microscope system and dye/light thrombogenesis method in mesenteric microvessels of rat dehydration model.
Materials and Methods: Five-week old male Wistar rats were used. 6 rats had free access to diet and water (control), 6 rats had free access to diet only (dehydration) for 24 hours. The rat was anesthetized with an injection of sodium pentobarbital into the femoral muscle. Rat mesentery was exposed on the observation stage according to the standard method. A venule with diameter of about 30 micro-meter was irradiated by the filtered light at 488 nm, followed by injection of a solution of 1.25% sodium fluorescein (2 mg/kg). The time taken from the irradiation to the start of the thrombus formation was recorded as the thrombus initiation time (Ti), and the time up to the complete stoppage of blood flow was recorded as the total occlusion time (Ts).
Results: Both Ti and Ts of dehydration group were significantly shortened compared with control group. Ti of dehydration group was one-third of control group, and Ts of dehydration group was one-half of control group.
Conclusion: The tendency of thrombogenesis is increased in dehydrate condition. It is thought effective rehydration method is very important in sport medicine.

PHT 3

PLATELET ACTIVATION AND PERIPHERAL ADRENERGIC/ SEROTONINERGIC IMPAIRMENT IN TYPE 2 DIABETES MELLITUS PATIENTS

F. Reis*, M.V. Campos*, L. Ruas, L. Almeida*, T. Alcobia*, M. Lourenço, A. Palmeiro, C.A. Ferrer-Antunes, M. Carvalheiro, F. Teixeira*
*Institute of Pharmacology and Experimental Therapeutics, Medicine Faculty, Coimbra University, 3004-504 Coimbra, Portugal

The study intended to evaluate some of the main cardiovascular risk indexes (haematology and lipid profile), the platelet activation as well as the peripheral sympathetic and serotoninergic nervous systems in a type 2 diabetes mellitus group (n=12) and in a sex-age-matched control group (n=7) of healthy volunteers. The study was ethically approved and subjects gave their consent. Results are means ± SEM (ANOVA and Fisher's test: *P<0.05; **P<0.01). Thrombin (0.5 U/ml)-evoked (by fura-2 fluorescence) intracellular Ca^{2+} release and transmembrane influx (156.7±8.0 ΛnM* and 192.3±10.2 ΛnM*) had a higher increase in the diabetic group vs control the (123.5±32.6; 147.8±4.1). PKC inhibition by staurosporin (0.1 μM) didn't have a significant influence on those $[Ca^{2+}]_i$ variations. ADP (2 μg/ml)-induced whole-blood platelet aggregation (impedance method) was higher in the diabetic group (16.2±2.9 ohms*) than in the control (8.4±1.7 ohms). The diabetic patients had lower plasma NA (423±49 pg/ml*) and AD (347±62 pg/ml) and platelet NA (226±76 pg/ml*) and AD (837±50 pg/ml) contents vs control (plasma: 858±103; 574±154; platelet: 457±34; 1119±132, respectively). Platelet 5-HT content was also lower in patients (5.0±0.7 ng/ml**) than in controls (32.1±6.5), while 5-HIAA was similar (all tested by HPLC-ECD). In conclusion, the type 2 diabetes group seems to be associated with peripheral sympathetic and serotoninergic systems impairment and platelet hyperactivation which might contribute to the increase risk of thromboembolic events and cardiovascular complications.

PHT 4

HEMORRHEOLOGICAL VARIABLES ASSOCIATED WITH INTIMA-MEDIA THICKNESS IN MYOCARDIAL INFARCTION PATIENTS

Oliveira V, Pedro AJ, Soares F., Batista P.
Neurological Department - Santa Maria Hospital - Lisbon Faculty of Medicine, Portugal

Introduction - Carotid Stenosis and Myocardial Infarction (MI) are manifestations of atherosclerosis in two territories. Intima Media Thickness (IMT) as measured by ultrasound duplex sonography, has been recognized as a marker for atherosclerosis and also hemorrheological parameters have been identified in association with atherosclerosis. We looked for associations between biochemical parameters and IMT in patients with acute MI.
Patients and Methods - 146 patients admitted to the Coronary Intensive Care Unit in our institution, during a 17 months period, with the diagnosis of acute MI were evaluated. All of them had carotid ultrasound examination including IMT assessment has described elsewhere. Blood samples were collected to determine values of Fibrinogen; Antithrombin III; t-PA 1; t-PA 2; PA-I; D-Dimer and Viscosity.
Results - Higher values of IMT were statistically associated with D-Dimer (r=0.33). There was a trend to the association with Fibrinogen (r=0.17), t-PA (r= -0.05) and Anti-thrombin III (r= -0.04).
Discusion – In our series of patients there was an association only with one parameter (D-Dimer). A trend with some others may due the relatively small number of patients. We may assume that a larger number of patients will lead to significance.
Conclusion - Higher values of IMT in patients with acute myocardial are associated with some hemorrheological parameters. A higher number of patients is necessary to confirm our results.

PHY 1

ENHANCED REACTIVE OXYGEN METABOLITE PRODUCTION IN LYMPHATICS OF SPONTANEOUSLY HYPERTENSIVE RATS

Frank A. DeLano and Geert W. Schmid-Schönbein
Microcirculation Laboratory, Department of Bioengineering, The Whitaker Institute for Biomedical Engineering, University of California, San Diego, La Jolla, California 92093-0412, U.S.A.

Hypertension is associated with a significantly increased risk for vascular lesions, microvascular complications and end organ failure. Among the hypotheses to account for the inflammation and enhanced organ injury may be an imbalance between reactive oxygen metabolite (ROM) generating and scavenging systems. No information exists about in-vivo mechanisms of ROM production for the lymphatic system in the spontaneously hypertensive rat (SHR). To explore the role of ROMs in the lymphatic system, localization of ROM production in rat mesenteric lymphatics was examined in mature normotensive Wistar Kyoto (WKY) rats and SHR. Tetranitroblue tetrazolium (TNBT), which in the presence of an oxidative challenge is reduced to colored insoluble formazans, was used to visualize oxidative stress. As an index of ROM formation, the optical density of the purple-black crystalline deposits (formazan) of reduced TNBT was measured on the endothelium which lines the wall of initial and collecting lymphatic vessels in mesentery using digital microscopy. Control measurements of ROMs in lymphatic vessels showed an readily detectable non-homogenous pattern of formazan deposits in both WKY and SHR. An enhanced level of ROM production was observed in lymphatic endothelium and lymphatic valves of SHR. These results indicate that compared with the normotensive WKY rats the level of ROMs is elevated in these lymphatics independent of the pressure elevation in the arterioles in the SHR. We also previously observed a similar rise of the ROMs in the venules of the SHR which also have no elevated blood pressure.
(Supported by NIH Grant HL-10881)

PHY 2

TRANSCRIPTION FACTORS AND THEIR CONTRIBUTION TO DOCA/SALT HYPERTENSION

AO Oyekan, MA Newaz, P Fidelis
Center for Cardiovascular Diseases, College of Pharmacy and Health Sciences, Texas Southern University, Houston TX 77004, USA

Peroxisome proliferator activated receptor α (PPARα), a ligand-activated transcription factor, mediates many cellular processes and protects against cardiovascular diseases, including hypertension. PPARα has been shown to increase nitric oxide (NO) and reduce endothelin-1 (ET-1) production via transcriptional regulation of their respective genes. Deoxycorticosterone acetate (DOCA)-salt hypertension is characterized by increased ET-1 and/or reduced NO production. This study tested the hypothesis that reduced PPARα expression/activity contributes to the pathogenesis of DOCA-salt hypertension and that PPARα activation exerts a protective effect in DOCA-salt hypertension via increased NO. DOCA (25 mg pellet s.c.) and 1-2% NaCl administration to uninephrectomized (Unx) mice led to markedly greater increases in systolic blood pressure (SBP; 190+10 vs 130+23 mmHg, $p<0.05$) and proteinuria (19+4 vs 8+4 mg/24 hr; $p<0.05$) in PPARα (-/-) than (+/+) mice. In UNx Sprague Dawley rats, DOCA administration reduced the expression of PPARα and medium-chain acylcoA dehydrogenase (MCAD), its downstream target gene, by 30 and 60%, respectively. Accompanying these was increased (SBP; 164+9 mmHg, p<005), protein excretion (3-fold), plasma ET-1 (28+5%, $p<0.05$) and reduced plasma NO (48+7%, $p<0.05$). Clofibrate (250 mg/kg/day; i.p), a PPARα ligand, reduced the elevated SBP to 125+12 mmHg ($p<0.05$), ET-1 (22+3%, $p<0.05$) and proteinuria (43±9%, $p<0.05$) and increased plasma and urinary NOx by 52±5% and 152±27% ($p<0.05$) respectively. Clofibrate also increased the expression of PPARα (78+15%, $p<0.05$) and MCAD (2-fold) protein and doubled PPARα activity (electrophoretic mobility shift assay) in the DOCA-salt rats. We conclude that reduced PPARα expression and activity contribute to increased ET-1 and reduced NO production in DOCA-salt hypertension and activation of PPARα may confer protection in this model of hypertension.

PIN 2

CD4+CD25+ REGULATORY T-CELLS ABROGATE HAPTEN-INDUCED LEUKO-CYTE/ENDOTHELIUM INTERACTION DURING CONTACT DERMATITIS: AN INTRAVITAL MICROSCOPIC STUDY IN AWAKE C57/BL6 MICE

S.C. SCHAEFER, S. RING[1], A. ENK[1], H.A. LEHR
Institute of Pathology, University Mainz
[1]Department of Dermatology, University Mainz, Germany

<u>Aims:</u> *In vitro* studies have indicated that the antiadhesive action of CD4+CD25+ T-cells requires cell-cell contact, presumably independent of cytokines. The exact mechanisms in vivo remain largely unknown. To study the role of CD4+CD25+ T-cells in a model of allergic contact dermatitis, we visualized the micro-circulatory changes directly at the site of inflammation using intravital fluorescence microscopy in awake mice. <u>Methods:</u> Dorsal skinfold chambers were chronically implanted into C57/BL6 mice, which allows visualization of leukocyte/endothelium inter-action in postcapillary venules. 6 days after sensitization with Trinitro-chlorbenzene (TNCB), FITC labeled CD4+CD25- or CD4+CD25+ T-cells were administered intravenously immediately prior to a second challenge with TNCB or carrier directly onto the skin side of the skinfold chamber. Through intravenous injection of the fluorescent marker Rhodamine, it was possible to differentiate endogenous, circulating leukocytes (Rho) and injected T-cells (FITC) during the subsequent inflammatory reaction. <u>Results:</u> Challenging with hapten caused a significant increase in slowly rolling and firmly adherent leukocytes within 4 hours. Injection of syngeneic CD4+CD25- T-cells did not influence the reaction pattern of allergic contact dermatitis whereas CD4+CD25+ regulatory T-cells entirely abrogated leukocyte/endothelium interaction and edema formation from the beginning. <u>Conclusion:</u> CD4+CD25+ regulatory T-cells prevent influx of effector T-cells during contact dermatitis. This points towards a novel mechanism by which regulatory T-cells modify immune reactions.

PIN 3

PHYSIOLOGICAL AND PATHOPHYSIOLOGICAL ROLES OF ANGIOTENSIN II IN THE RAT SYNOVIUM

A. G. Price[1], J.C. Lockhart[1], W.R. Ferrell[2]
[1]Biological Sciences, University of Paisley, Paisley, PA1 2BE, UK;
[2]Centre for Rheumatic Diseases, Royal Infirmary, Glasgow, G31 2ER, UK.

Angiotensin II (Ang II) is classically known as a potent vasoconstrictor in the systemic circulation, but its role(s) in the joint requires elucidation. Adult male Wistar rats (350 ± 20 g b.wt., mean ± SEM, n=6) were anaesthetised using 25% urethane and an ellipse of skin overlying the joint removed. The carotid artery was cannulated to enable monitoring of blood pressure. Synovial perfusion was measured using a laser Doppler imager (Moor Instruments Ltd, Axminster, UK). Scans were taken after 0.1 ml topical administration of saline then sequentially after increasing concentrations of the desired drug. Topical application of Ang II (10^{-16} mol – 10^{-9} mol) produced biphasic vascular effects: vasodilating at low doses (10^{-16} – 10^{-13} mol) and vasoconstricting at high doses (10^{-12} – 10^{-9} mol). Topical losartan (10^{-12} – 10^{-7} mol; Merck & Co, USA) alone was further used to assess the vascular role of endogenous Ang II. The resulting decreases in flux suggest that endogenous Ang II may act as a vasodilator in maintaining synovial blood flow ($P<0.015$; one-way ANOVA; n=6-8). We further examined the role of Ang II in Freunds adjuvant-induced (FCA) chronic joint inflammation by subcutaneous injection of 15 mg/kg losartan prophylactically with maintenance doses every 2 days; a vehicle-treated inflamed group was included as control. Joint swelling was assessed by measurement of joint diameter using callipers and expressed as percentage change from pre-induction values. The established joint swelling at day 14 (65.8 ± 1.9%; n=4) was significantly ($P<0.0001$; t-test) and substantially reduced by losartan treatment (16.9 ± 3.5%; n=4). Western blot analysis demonstrated substantial upregulation of AT_1 receptors in FCA rats. These data suggest Ang II has both physiological and pathophysiological roles in the joint.

PIN 4

INHIBITION OF PAR-2 ACTIVATION ATTENUATES ACUTE JOINT INFLAMMATION

E.B. Kelso[1], L. Dunning[2], J.C. Lockhart[2], W.R.. Ferrell[1], M.D. Hollenberg[3]
[1]Centre for Rheumatic Diseases, University of Glasgow, Glasgow, G31 2ER, UK; [2]Biological Sciences, University of Paisley, Paisley, PA1 2BE, UK; [3]Department of Pharmacology, University of Calgary, Alberta, Canada.

We recently demonstrated a substantially attenuated inflammatory response to Freund's complete adjuvant in proteinase-activated receptor-2 (PAR-2) 'knock-out' mice [Ferrell WR et al J. Clin Invest.111 35-41]. The present study investigated whether PAR-2 presents a new therapeutic target in arthritis by using a polyclonal antibody (B5) to the trypsin-binding site on PAR-2 in a murine model of acute inflammation. Knee joint inflammation was induced by intra-articular injection of carrageenan/kaolin (CK) mixture (20μl) in deeply anaesthetised male C57BL/6J mice (n=6). In a parallel group (n=6), B5 (20μl) was co-administered by intra-articular injection prior to injection of CK. A further group (n=6) were pre-treated with non-immune serum. Swelling was measured 24 hours post-induction using callipers and expressed as % of pre-injection values. The volume of fluid injected does not cause measurable joint swelling. CK alone resulted in a 25.9 ± 3.6% (mean ± SEM) increase in joint diameter at 24 hours that was significantly attenuated ($P < 0.002$) by intra-articular co-administration of the B5 antibody (6.4 ± 2.5%). Non-immune serum gave a response (20.2 ± 4.2%) that did not differ significantly (P=0.36) from that obtained with CK.

This fourfold reduction of joint inflammation suggests that inhibition of PAR-2 activation has anti-inflammatory potential. This result confirms and extends our earlier findings in PAR-2 'knockout' mice, supporting the concept of PAR-2 as a therapeutic target for future studies in models of arthritis. [Arthritis Research Campaign Grant L0559]

PIN 5

SYNOVIAL PERFUSION AND COX-2 INHIBITION

J.S. McLean[1], L. Dunning[1], J.C. Lockhart[1], W.R. Ferrell[2]
[1]Biological Sciences, University of Paisley, Paisley, PA1 2BE and [2]Centre for Rheumatic Diseases Glasgow Royal Infirmary, Glasgow, G31 2ER, Scotland, United Kingdom.

Basal synovial perfusion is dependent on the prostanoid system as administration of the broad-spectrum cyclooxygenase (COX) inhibitor results in increased vascular resistance [Najafipour H. & Ferrell W.R. Expt. Physiol. 1994; 79: 93-101]. This study used a selective COX-2 inhibitor, MF-Tricyclic (Merck & Co, USA), to dissect out the relative involvement of COX-1 and COX-2 in the regulation of synovial perfusion.

Male Wistar rats were deeply anaesthetized using 25% urethane and all procedures were performed in accordance with current UK regulations. Blood pressure was monitored continuously via carotid artery cannulation and knee joint perfusion assessed using a laser Doppler imager (Moor Instruments Ltd, Axminster, UK). Indomethacin or MF-Tricyclic, were administered by intravenous infusion (both at 3mg/ml).

Indomethacin administration resulted in a progressive increase in joint vascular resistance by approximately 60% over a 40 minute period (P = 0.001; two-way ANOVA) whereas MF-Tricyclic infusion did not significantly change resistance, being similar to infusion of vehicle.

These results suggest that basal synovial perfusion is dependent on COX-1, the constitutive form of cyclo-oxygenase, and not on COX-2 which is induced during inflammatory responses. This indicates that, apart from their adavantage in giving rise to fewer serious gastro-intestinal side effects, COX-2 inhibitors such as MF-Tricyclic may also maintain joint perfusion, thereby preventing synovial hypoxia which is known to occur in inflamed joints and which may contribute to the pathogenesis of arthritis.

PIN 6

VASCULAR ENDOTHELIAL CONTROL OF THE CIRCULATING INFLAMMATORY MEDIATOR XANTHINE OXIDOREDUCTASE

J. Hewinson, C.R. Stevens, M. Horrocks, & T.M. Millar.
School for Health, University of Bath, Bath, BA2 7AY, England.

Xanthine oxidoreductase (XOR) catalyses the production of reactive oxygen and nitrogen species (RONS). XOR is found in the liver, mammary gland, and pancreas at high levels, and also circulates. The circulating form has been associated with endothelial dysfunction and inflammatory diseases such as acute respiratory distress syndrome (ARDS). Limited studies have shown that the vascular endothelium may release and endocytose XOR. We propose the endothelium is an important site for controlling circulating XOR and aim to characterise the mechanisms for XOR release and endocytosis from this site.

Using cultured human umbilical vein endothelial cells (HUVECs) as an endothelial model (with ethical approval), the release and uptake of XOR were assessed. XOR activity was measured using a sensitive fluorescence-based assay and XOR protein was detected using immunofluorescence and flow cytometry.

HUVEC XOR exhibits a punctate, cytoplasmic stain independent of von Willebrand factor storage. Using the known endothelial cell stimulators histamine and thrombin, we have demonstrated a significantly higher release of XOR compared to controls ($p<0.001$). In addition, thrombin significantly increased XOR activity in a dose-dependent manner, a proteolytic process may be responsible. The endocytosis of XOR by the vascular endothelium was demonstrated.

We have demonstrated a mechanism for inducing localised endothelial XOR release and capture that could contribute to free radical damage both locally and systemically. This mechanism may be responsible for ARDS and vascular damage associated with RONS.

PIN 7

TOLL LIKE RECEPTOR 4 AND COMPLEMENT BOTH CONTRIBUTE TO THE LOCALISED SHWARTZMAN REACTION IN MICE.

M.Ali, K.E.Norman.
Cardiovascular research unit, Cnical scíences department, The University of Sheffield, Herries Road, sheffield, S5 7 AU. UK.

Cellular responses to the bacterial cell walJ product lipopolysaccharide (LPS) require Toll-like receptor 4 (TLR4) and mice lacking functional TLR4 are protected from the hannful effects ofthis agent. LPS also activates the complement cascade and does so in the absence ofTLR4 and other cenular components. The localised Shwartzman reactíon (LSR) is a model of dissemínated intravascular coagulation that develops following two injections ofLPS and is dependent on both complement and inflammatory cell activation. We have explored contributions ofTLR4 and complement to the pathology associated with the LSR in mice. C57BL/6 mice were injected with TNF-a (500ng, intrascrotalJy) 4 h prior to surgery. Intravital microscopy was then performed and LPS was injected (i.v). LSR development was studied in a network of post capillary venules for up to 1 h after LPS injection. Total vessel area, leukocyte aggregate area, and the number haemorrhages were determined before and every 10 minutes after treatment. Leukocyte aggregation was observed in post-capillary venules ofTNF-a primed mice within 10 minutes ofLPS administration and peaked at 30 minutes. Haemorrhagic injury peaked 40 minutes after LPS and did not co-Iocalise with sites of leukocyte aggregation. C3H/HeJ (LPS resistant) mice had reduced aggregation and no haemorrhage compared to controI mice (C3H/He1\T). C3H/HeJ mice transplanted with C3H/HeN bone malTOW also had reduced aggregation implicating leukocyte TLR4 in the response to LPS in the LSR. Cobra venom factor treated mice did not develop aggregates or haemorrhage, confinning complement dependence ofthe LSR.

PIN 8

CHANNEL BLOCKING DURING THE FLOW OF WHOLE BLOOD THROUGH AN ARRAY OF CAPILLARY-SIZE MICROCHANNELS BY LEUKOCYTES EXPOSED TO *MYCOPLASMA* LIPOPROTEIN (LPSAL) AND E. COLI LPS

Y. Kikuchi*, H. E. Kikuchi, T. Miyake, N. Mizukami, T. Kurosu, K. Ogoshi, and K. Shibata
Department of Oral Pathological Science, Graduate School of Dental Medicine, Hokkaido University, Sapporo 060-0813, *Microchannel Array Technology Team, National Food Research Institute, Tsukuba 305-8642, Japan

Role of microcirculatory blood rheology is still not well understood in the occurrence of multiple organ failure in sepsis. Recently, microfabricated channel arrays have been used for studies of rheological events in the microcirculation both under physiological and pathological conditions. The present report studied capillary blocking by leukocytes activated by bacterial stimulation.
Heparinized whole blood samples were obtained from 24 healthy volunteers and an aliquot of each whole blood sample was caused to flow through a microchannel array (width 7 micron, depth 4.5 micron, length 30 micron, number 8736 in parallel) under 20 cmH2O pressure difference with the addition of *Mycoplasma salivarium* lipoprotein (LPsal; final concentration 400 ng/ml - 4 micro-g/ml)) and *E. coli* LPS (final concentration 2 ng/ml – 2 micro-g/ml). The transit time was determined for each 10 micro-l whole blood to flow from 0 to 100 micro-l. The microchannel blocking rate was calculated by (1 – transit time (0-10 micro-l)/transit time (90-100 micro-l)) x 100. The microchannel blocking took place to a various extent even for control whole blood and its rate showed a correlation with both systolic and diastolic blood pressures. The rate increased in a dose dependent manner with the addition of LPsal and LPS; different subjects showed considerably different sensitivities in the response. The blocking rate became largest at 30 min after the exposure.

PIN 9

REGULATION OF NEUTROPHIL APOPTOSIS DURING THE ACUTE INFLAMMATORY RESPONSE: DIFFERENTIAL INVOLVEMNET OF BAX-α AND BAD

P. Weinmann and B. Walzog
Dept. of Physiology, Ludwig-Maximilians-Universität, 80336 Munich, Germany.

The control of neutrophil apoptosis plays an important role in homeostasis and inflammation. Using intraperitoneal injection of thioglycollate in mice as a model for an aseptic inflammatory response, we found that apoptosis of isolated blood PMN was markedly impaired within 4 h of culture from 27.0% in PMN derived from untreated control mice to 17.2% in PMN isolated from the blood of mice with acute peritonitis as measured by detecting the loss of DNA content. This finding was confirmed by detecting the down-regulation of CD16 expression in whole blood samples. Extravasated PMN that were collected from the peritoneal cavity of mice with acute peritonitis showed an almost 2-fold increase of apoptosis, when compared to inflammatory blood PMN as measured by detecting the loss of DNA content. This finding was confirmed by detecting the condensation of the nuclei by acridine orange staining. In contrast, no significant difference of PMN apoptosis was observed in PMN derived from the bone marrow of mice with or without peritonitis. Whereas the observed delay of apoptosis in inflammatory blood PMN was associated with a decrease of Bax-α protein expression, the enhancement of apoptosis in extravasated PMN was accompanied by an up-regulation of Bad. Taken together, these findings suggest that PMN apoptosis in blood and tissue is differentially regulated during the inflammatory response via Bax-α and Bad, two proapoptotic members of the Bcl-2 family of apoptosis-associated genes. (Supported by SFB 366/C3)

PIN 10

TRYPSIN-INDUCED NEUTROPHIL DEGRANULATION AND MATRIX METALLOPROTEINASE-9 ACTIVATION – A TIME-FRAME ANALYSIS.

H.S. Rosario, C. Saldanha, J. Martins-Silva
Institute of Biochemistry, Faculty of Medicine of Lisbon and Vascular Pathobiology Unit, Institute of Molecular Medicine, Lisbon, Portugal.

We have previously demonstrated that pancreatic trypsin plays a proinflammatory role in acute intestinal ischemia-reperfusion, namely increasing neutrophil infiltration into the intestinal wall. In the same setting, trypsin was shown to acutely activate neutrophil-released matrix metalloproteinase-9 (MMP-9), in a process that can contribute to the intense morphological injury and inflammation present in intestinal ischemia-reperfusion. To clarify these *in vivo* findings, we aimed at studying the *in vitro* dynamics of trypsin-induced activation of proMMP-9 released from degranulated neutrophils.

Human neutrophils were isolated from peripheral venous blood and activated with proinflammatory phorbol myristate acetate (PMA) or with different concentrations of pancreatic trypsin. Aliquots from the supernatant were collected at different intervals, and the amount of MMP-9 (either proform or active form) released by the neutrophils was assessed by gelatin zymography.

The results show that trypsin plays a significant role as activator of MMP-9 released by neutrophils stimulated with PMA. This process of proMMP-9 activation occurs very rapidly following the release of MMP-9. We also show that trypsin itself induces neutrophil activation, in a process that occurs almost simultaneously to MMP-9 activation.

We conclude that pancreatic trypsin may play a dual role in the development of the neutrophil-dependent inflammatory response in the intestinal wall, both as cell activator and a positive modulator of proinflammatory MMP-9 as it is released by the degranulating neutrophil.

PIR 1

CHANGES OF THE TOTAL ANTIOXIDANT POTENTIAL IN BLOOD SERUM OF ACUTE MYOCARDIAL INFARCTION PATIENTS TREATED BY FIBRYNOLYSIS OR ANGIOPLASTY

R. Gil[2], B.K. Glód[1], P. Grieb[1], T. Kulawik[2], A. Wozniak[1],
[1]Department of Experimental Pharmacology, Medical Research Center, Polish Academy of Sciences, ul. Pawi_skiego 5, 03-187 Warsaw, Poland
[2]Central Clinical Hospital Ministry of Internal Affairs and Administra-tion, Clinic of Cardiology, ul. Wo_oska 137, 02-507 Warsaw, Poland

The only effective treatment of acute myocardial infarction (AMI) is based on a quick induction of reperfusion in the infarcted coronary artery.
The two procedures most frequently employed to induce coronary reperfusion are systemic fibrynolitic treatment (SFT) and percutaneous angioplasty (PTCA). Furthermore, since some major side effects of quick coronary reperfusion (such as myocardial stunning) are related to the activation of free radical generation in cardiac tissues, supplementation of reperfusion treatment of AMI with low molecular weight antioxidants such as N-acetylcysteine (NAC) has been considered. Serum total antioxidant potential (TAP) is the measure blood ability to inactivate free radicals. The aims of the present study were to: a) describe and compare the changes in serum TAP which occur over 24 hrs after post-AMI reperfusion produced by SFT or PTCA, and b) to find out whether intravenous treatment with NAC (7.2 g over 24 h) will modify changes of TAP which occur following SFT. Surprisingly we have found that plasma TAP transiently increases following coronary reperfusion. This effect, independent of the treatment modality (SFT or PTCA),was caused by increase of TAP associated with plasma proteins. However, no correlation of TAP was found with either total protein, or C-reactive protein level. No correlation was also found between TAP and LVdD, EF and LVEdD at 3 months. We also have found that treatment with NAC did not influence TAP, although it seemed to decrease peak CPK slightly.

PIR 2

RAT CREMASTER MUSCLE TRANSPLANTATION AFTER COLD STORAGE: EVALUATION OF CAPILLARY PERFUSION

J. Bastiaanse[1], D.W. Slaaf[2], L.V. Nanhekhan[1], W.D. Boeckx[1], M.G.A. oude Egbrink[3]
[1]Dept of Plastic and Reconstructive Surgery, University Hospital Maastricht, P.O. Box 5800, 6202 AZ Maastricht,. Cardiovascular Research Institute Maastricht, Depts of [2]Biophysics and [3]Physiology, Maastricht University, P.O. Box 616, 6200 MD Maastricht, The Netherlands.

Ischemia/reperfusion injury (IRI) is often the final and irreversible factor causing flap failure in microvascular surgery for reconstruction of complex defects. The aim of this study was to assess the feasibility of cremaster transplantation in rats and to investigate effects of cold storage in a preservation solution on IRI.
Cremaster transplantations were performed immediately (n=6), or after a period of 8 or 24 hours of cold storage in the preservation solution HTK (n=12) or in saline (n=12). Data were compared to a control group (no transplantation). Intravital microscopy was used to quantify capillary perfusion during an observation period of 3 hours following transplantation. The transplantation procedure itself causes an ischemic period of 60 minutes. After direct transplantation (without cold preservation), only a slight decrease in capillary perfusion to 90% of control values was observed. Transplantation after 8 hours of cold storage in HTK resulted in an increase in capillary perfusion to 112% compared to control ($p<0.01$). After 24 h cold storage in HTK, perfusion was still 75-80% of control values. Storage in saline (24h) resulted in low capillary perfusion after transplantation (40% of control values; $p<0.01$).
Capillary perfusion is well preserved after transplantation of rat cremaster muscle after 8 or 24 h of cold storage in HTK. Cold storage in saline did not preserve cremaster capillary perfusion in this transplantation model.

PIR 3

INTRALUMINAL PANCREATIC TRYPSIN INCREASES NEUTROPHIL INFILTRATION INTO THE INTESTINAL WALL DURING ACUTE ISCHEMIA-REPERFUSION

H.S. Rosario[1,2], S.W. Waldo[1], G.W. Schmid-Schönbein[1]
[1]Dept of Bioengineering, University of California San Diego, La Jolla, CA; [2]Institute of Biochemistry, Faculty of Medicine of Lisbon and Vascular Pathobiology Unit, Institute of Molecular Medicine, Lisbon, Portugal.

Intraluminal pancreatic enzymes, namely trypsin, are associated with morphological damage in intestinal ischemia-reperfusion. This study was performed to investigate if trypsin can also modulate the neutrophil-dependent inflammation associated with ischemia-reperfusion.
To achieve this purpose we developed a surgical technique in the rat, in which a single jejunal loop was isolated and connected to an intraluminal perfusion system with Krebs-Henseleit buffer (3 mL/min). The animals were divided in an ischemia-reperfusion group, by clamping the vascular supply to the loop for 45 minutes and then reperfusing it for 90 minutes; and a control group. In half of the animals from each group the perfusion buffer was supplemented with trypsin (1 mg/mL). Leukocyte-endothelial interaction was analysed in the intestinal wall with intravital microscopy. In different animals, the jejunal loop was collected and cryosections were obtained for histology, histochemistry for neutrophilic myeloperoxidase and immunofluorescent detection of neutrophils.
Venular leukocyte rolling and adhesion was increased in the ischemia-reperfusion group with intraluminal trypsin, compared to controls and ischemia-reperfusion without trypsin. The different histological techniques applied consistently showed a heavy inflammatory infiltrate into the intestinal wall consisting mostly of neutrophils.
These results suggest that pancreatic trypsin present in the lumen of the intestine plays a role in the acute inflammatory response and neutrophil infiltration that follows intestinal ischemia-reperfusion.
Supported by HL 67825 and FLAD 470/2000.

POF 1

CLOZAPINE DIRECTLY RELAXES BOVINE RETINAL ARTERIES

J. Van de Voorde, K. Boussery, S. Lambrecht, C. Delaey
Department of Physiology and Pathophysiology, Ghent University,
De Pintelaan 185, 9000 Gent, Belgium.

It has been suggested that the atypical antipsychotic drug clozapine might be helpful in the development of new antiglaucoma agents, since it combines lowering of the intra-ocular pressure after topical instillation with vasodilation. However, the vasoactive influence of clozapine on ocular blood vessels has never been analysed. Therefore, this study aimed to evaluate whether clozapine has direct vasodilatory effects in isolated bovine retinal arteries (BRA) and to characterise pharmacologically the mechanisms involved.

Retinal arteries were isolated from bovine eyes and mounted in a wire-myograph for isometric tension recording. Concentration-response curves were generated by cumulative addition of clozapine (1 nM to 10 μM) to the organ bath.

Clozapine elicited a concentration-dependent relaxation of the BRA. Removal of the endothelium of the BRA, inhibition of nitric oxide synthase with N^{ω}-nitro-L-arginine and inhibition of soluble guanylyl cyclase with ODQ (1H-[1,2,4]oxadiazolo[4,3-a]quinoxalin-1-one) significantly attenuated the clozapine-response, whereas cyclo-oxygenase inhibition with indomethacin had no influence. The Ca^{2+} channel activator Bay k8644, the nonselective 5-hydroxytryptamine receptor antagonist methiothepin and the adenosine receptor antagonist 8-(p-sulfophenyl) theophylline also failed in affecting the clozapine-induced relaxations.

In conclusion, clozapine clearly relaxes bovine retinal arteries in a direct way. Endothelium-derived NO is involved in this response. However, prostanoids, calcium entry blockade, $5\text{-}HT_7$ receptor stimulation and adenosine receptor stimulation all seem to be not involved.

POP 1

LASER DOPPLER FLOWMETRY IN SICKLE CELL PATIENTS WITH AND WITHOUT HYDROXYREA.

Amaal El BEshlawy, Mona El Tagy, Aly El Ashmaoui, , Eman Abdel Raouf and Ireny Fawzy. From the department of Pediatrics and Medicine, Cairo University, Egypt

Laser Doppler flowmetry (LDPM) was done for 55 Sickle cell disease patients (SCD) who were attending the Hematology Clinic, Children Hospital, Cairo University comparable with both 11 normal controls and 11 B thalassemia patients. We followed up our patients every 6 months by LDPM. Patients were divided into cases on Hydroxyurea (24 cases) and cases on conservative treatment with repeated blood transfusion (28 cases). The basal blood flow of skin microcirculation by LDPM was significantly higher in SCD patients than normal controls and thalassemia patients. The time to peak in both thermal and reactive hyperemia tests were significantly prolonged in SCD patients than normal controls and thalassemia patients. The percent changes after both thermal stimulation and post reactive hyperemia tests were lower in SCD than normal controls and thalassemia. SCD patients exhibited higher frequencies and powers of the basal vasomotions as well as the post thermal and post reactive hyperemia vasomotions than normal controls and thalassemia patients. During follow up, SCD patients on HU showed significant reduction of the basal blood flow than those on conservative treatment. They also showed significant improvement of the time to peak in both thermal and reactive hyperemia tests when compared with those on conservative treatment. The percent changes after thermal stimulation and reactive hyperemia were significantly higher in patients on HU than those on conservative treatment SCD patients on HU showed improvement of their vasomotions than those on conservative treatment. It was concluded that Laser Doppler flowmetry is a sensitive and reliable technique in the follow up of SCD and might help to guide therapy and assess prognosis.

POP 2

MICROVASCULAR CHANGES OF GENGIVAL TISSUE AFTER ULTRASONIC TOOTH PREPARATION

M. Matsuo and K. Tamaki
Institute for Frontier Oral Science and Prosthodontics, Kanagawa Dental College, Yokosuka, 2388580, Kanagawa, Japan.

Tooth preparation is one of the important process in dental treatment. Accuracy in this process is greatly influenced by the type of preparatory instruments used, the proficiency of the dentist and the anatomical shape of tooth. If it is not done properly, it is possible to damage the teeth and gingival tissue. In this study, we examined the influence of changes in gingival microcirculation after tooth preparation using ultrasonic waves.

Molars with beagle dogs were used. Preparation was carried out with a ultrasonic wave instruments along the height of the gingival margin. As a control, the same size and structure of a conventional diamond bar was used with the dental air turbine. The micro vascular resin cast model was made, synthetic resin was injected from the alveolar arteries and peripheral tissues were dissolved with a 10% Hcl and 15% KOH solution. These specimens were examined under a scanning electron microscope (SEM).

In the ultrasonic preparation group, the vasculature closely resembles healthy gingiva and in the dental turbine group, the vascular network of the sulcular epithelium changed into a dilated renal glomerulus-like form. The injected vascular resin leaked out from the blood vessels beneath the epithelium. The leakage of the resin from the blood vessels was observed in the dental turbine group, which means not only the destruction of blood vessels but also that the endothelial cell gap opens by hyper permeability in the attached epithelium area. In the ultrasonic preparation, the blood vessels did not changed and the vasculature showed a form equal to the healthy gingiva. These results suggest that preparation by ultrasonic instruments minimizes damage to the gingival tissue.

POP 3

THE QTc PEAK INTERVAL DISPERSION IN PATIENTS WITH HYPERTHYROIDIA AND SYSTEMIC HYPERTENSION

S.Tudorica,C.Tudorica*,M. Moise**,M. Muraru*, D.Spataru*,A.Stoica***
"Masina de Paine" Endocrinology Ambulatory,*Coltea Clinical Hospital, ** Diagnostic and Treatment Center " Dr.Victor Babes",***Medicover Center, Bucharest, Romania

Objective: the analyse of QTc peak interval dispersion in patients with hyperthyroidia for more than two years,in treatment permanently maintained with βblockers and antithyroidian agents. Material:140 patients medium age 47,5 years; sex ratio M/F:4/3; the average duration of hyperthyroidia 3 years; normal values of T3,T4 and TSH at this moment.They were divided into two groups: the control group - 65 normal subjects and the study groups - 75 hyperthyroidian patients Method: retrospective study; T3, T4 and TSH values, standard ECG (manually measurement of QT peak interval, the correction with Bazet formula, the calculation of QT peak dispersion), transthoracic echocardiography M, 2D - mode and Doppler for left ventricular function evaluation (ejection fraction-EF; shortening fraction-SF; E/A peak velocities; isovolumic relaxation time-IVRT, LV mass). Exclusion criteria: valvulopaties, LV mass>125g/m2, atrioventricular conduction disturbances, recent symptoms of hyperthyroidia, increased values of T3, T4, TSH, heart rate > 110 beats/min or < 60 beats/min, drugs that altered QT interval duration or dispersion, bundle branch blocks. Results: the average value of QTc peak dispersion was 54,1 (3,4) ms in study group and 48,6 (4,8)ms in control group. Conclusion: all the investigated patients had a normal left ventricular mass and function. In hyperthyroidian patients regardless of β-blocker therapy the left ventricular function, QTc peak was within normal limits. It is likely that these patients have a high cardiovascular risk only in the late phases, consecutively of LV mass augmentation and structural alteration of the myofibriles.

POP 4

REMODELING OF CAPILLARY NETWORK AND TUNEL POSITIVE ENDOTHELIUM IN HINDLIMB UNWEIGHTED ATROPHIED SOLEUS MUSCLE

H. Fujino,[1,2] H. Kohzuki,[1,3] H Tasaki,[2] I. Takeda,[2] and F. Kajiya[1]
[1]Department of Cardiovascular Physiology, Okayama University Graduate School of Medicine and Dentistry, Okayama, Okayama 700-8558
[2]Department of Physical Therapy, Suzuka University of Medical Science, Suzuka, Mie 510-0293
[3]Department of Food and Nutrition, Okayama Gakuin University, Kurashiki, Okayama 710-8511, Japan

Little is known regarding three-dimensional architecture changes in skeletal muscle capillaries with hindlimb unweighting induced muscle atrophy. In this study, we focused on structural alterations of the capillary network, especially intercapillary anastomosis, vascular apoptosis and tortuosity in the soleus muscle of rats after 2wks of hindlimb unweighting (HU). Detailed three-dimensional architecture of capillary network of perfusion-fixed specimen was visualized using confocal laser scanning microscope. The mean capillary volume, capillary toutuosity, the number of intercapillary anastomosis and capillary luminal diameter were significantly smaller in HU than in age-matched control. Increased TUNEL positive endothelial cells were recognized in atrophied soleus, indicating negative angiogenesis in the atrophied muscle, e.g., pruning and decreased cell number. These results indicate that muscle atrophy by HU generates microstructural alterations of capillary network, and apoptosis occurs remarkable in intercapillary endothelial cell of the anastomoses and/or tortuous capillaries.

POP 5

TESTING FOR RAYNAUD'S PHENOMENON UTILIZING LASER DOPPLER FLUX (LDF) AND AMBIENT WARMING

P.W. Wennberg, D.A. Liedl, T.W. Rooke, R.F.J. Shepherd
Gonda Vascular Center and Division of Cardiovascular Disease, Mayo Clinic, Rochester MN, 55906, USA

Purpose--Primary Raynaud's phenomenon (RP) is a common benign condition. Secondary RP may be associated with disease processes with arteropathy. Ice water immersion with rewarming time or macrovascular changes on Duplex ultrasound has been used to test RP. We sought to develop a method to differentiate primary from secondary RP wihtout cold exposure utilizing LDF and response to warming.

Methods—256 patients over 18 months were referred for evaluation of RP. Complete evaluation consisted of segmental pressures including fingers, pulse volume recording, Doppler signals and resting temperatures. We obtained baseline LDF values (Periflux 5000, Perimed, Sweden) with and unheated probe at each digit. Patients with finger temperatures less than 30C were warmed in a 45C incubator for 20 minutes and LDF again recorded, now with a heated probe. 53 patients underwent angiography allowing comparison of a "gold standard" for occlusive disease.

Results—33 of 53 patients had occlusive disease on angiography. LDF at baseline did not correlate with the presence or absence of occlusive disease. In patients without occlusive disease, LDF value of greater than 200 units following warming indicated a normal response (primary RP). Failure to increase LDF with warming, or, more so a fall in LDF with warming indicated presence of occlusive disease (secondary RP). There was one false positive and one fase negative. Sensitivity and specificity of the method are both greater than 95%.

Conclusion—LDF at baseline and following ambient warming is a sensitive and specific method for differentiation of primary from secondary RP. The non-invasive methodology makes it an excellent screening tool.

POP 6

PLASMA VISCOSITY AND ERYTHROCYTE DEFORMABILITY IN OBSTRUCTIVE SLEEP APNEA SYNDROME

E.Ileri, N.Dikmenoglu, N. Seringec, B. Ciftci, S.F. Guven
Dept. of Physiology, Hacettepe University, Ankara, 06100, Turkey

Obstructive Sleep Apnea Syndrome (OSAS) is characterized by repeated obstructions of the upper respiratory tract during sleep. Myocardial infarctions and strokes happen more frequently in OSAS patients and cardiovascular problems occur frequently during morning hours. Blood viscosity has been reported to increase during morning hours in OSAS patients. However the parameters that make up blood viscosity have not been studied in detail. The present study aimed to examine in OSAS patients, two of the parameters that influence blood viscosity: plasma viscosity and erythrocyte deformability.

11 patients with severe OSAS (8M-3F; age = 50.18 ± 8.06; apnea-hypopnea index, AHI = 55.2 ± 24.53; BMI = 31.06 ± 3.71) and 11 healthy nonsmoking volunteers of similar sex, age and BMI were studied. The study was approved by the local ethics committee and patients gave written informed consent. Venous blood samples were obtained twice a day: in the morning (08:30-09:00 a.m.) and in the evening (16:30-17:30 p.m.). Erythrocyte deformability was studied by filtration method and plasma viscosity was studied by cone-plate viscometer.

OSAS patients had a higher plasma viscosity in the morning ($p<0.05$) and both morning and evening values were higher than controls ($p<0.05$). No morning and evening changes were observed in controls. No ertythrocyte deformability changes were observed between patients and controls. Hct, MCV and MCHC values were not changed in patients either.

We conclude that the plasma viscosity, even lower in the evening, is higher in severe OSAS patients. This condition results with an increase in whole blood viscosity and it may contribute to the increased incidence of cardiovascular events in OSAS patients in the morning.

POP 7

PHYTOSTEROLS IN MILK EFFECTS ON PLASMA CHOLESTEROL CONCENTRATIONS: EXPERIMENTAL EVIDENCE IN PORTUGUESE HEALTHY SUBJECTS

S. Gonçalves, A. S. Silva, C. Branco, C. Saldanha, J. Martins e Silva
Instituto de Bioquímica, Faculdade de Medicina de Lisboa, Unidade de Biopatologia Vascular, Instituto de Medicina Molecular, 1649-028 Lisboa, Portugal.

Cholesterol is important for the body's functions. It contributes to cell membranes configuration and properties and in synthesis of certain hormones. Absorbable cholesterol comes from three sources: the diet, the liver and from intestinal cell turnover. Artery-clogging plaques may be formed from excess of plasma cholesterol levels, increasing vascular event. Plant phytosterols are known to suppress intestinal cholesterol absorption even through the mechanisms has not been established. The present study investigated the effects of phytosterols-milk in take in plasma cholesterol levels. Twenty healthy subjects were fed a milk-sterol containing (2mg/day) for thirty days. The subjects were instructed to maintain the same dietary intake during the study. Concentrations of total cholesterol, HDL-cholesterol and LDL-cholesterol were measured in the beginning, after fifteen days and thirty days of phytosterols intake. After fifteen days of treatment total cholesterol and LDL-cholesterol concentrations were decreased significantly by 9%; $p < 0.05$ and 11.48%; $p < 0.05$, respectively. After thirty days, the values did not change significantly in relation with the results obtained at fifteen days. These results show a decrease in plasma cholesterol levels with a drinking diet enriched with phytosterols with concentrations of sterols much lower as reported before.

POP 8

PHYTOSTEROLS IN MILK AS A DEPRESSOR OF PLASMA CHOLESTEROL LEVELS: EXPERIMENTAL EVIDENCE IN HYPERCHOLESTEROLEMIC SUBJECTS

S. Gonçalves1, A. S. Silva[1], C. Saldanha[1], J. Martins e Silva[1], A. V. Maria[2]
[1]Instituto de Bioquímica, Faculdade de Medicina de Lisboa, Unidade de Biopatologia Vascular, Instituto de Medicina Molecular, 1649-028 Lisboa Portugal.
[2]Instituto de Medicina Preventiva, Faculdade de Medicina, 1649-028 Lisboa Portugal.

Cholesterol is a fatty substance that forms deposits in the blood vessel. Artery-clogging plaques may formed when among others factors, cholesterol levels become too high, so blood vessels become blocked and are unable to supply blood to the heart or brain, triggering a heart attack or stroke. Vegetal sterols have been reported to decreased plasma concentrations of cholesterol without any side effects. In order to evaluate if milk should be a good vehicle for phytosterols lowering cholesterol plasma levels, we performed a study of thirty hypercholesterolemic patients (LDL-cholesterol > 130mg/dL) treated with enriched phytosterols milk (2g/day). Hypercholesterolemic patients of match age and sex drinking equal type of milk but without phytosterols were used as control group. The subjects were instructed to maintain the same dietary intake during the study. Concentrations of total cholesterol, HDL-cholesterol and LDL-cholesterol were measured in the beginning, after fifteen and thirty days of milk beverage. After fifteen days of treatment total cholesterol and LDL-cholesterol concentrations were decreased significantly by 10.08%; $p < 0.05$ and 12.74%; $p < 0.05$, respectively. After thirty days, the values did not change significantly in relation with the results obtained at fifteen days. These results show a positive effect with the milk as a good food vehicle as lowering plasma cholesterol in the treatment of hypercholesterolemia.

POP 9

EFFECTS OF PHYTOSTEROLS SUPPLIED IN HALF-FAT AND LOW-FAT MILK, IN THE PLASMA CHOLESTEROL CONCENTRATIONS IN RATS

AS. Silva, C. Branco, J. Martins e Silva, C. Saldanha
Instituto de Bioquímica, Faculdade de Medicina de Lisboa, Unidade de Biopatologia Vascular, IMM 1649-028 Lisboa, Portugal

Clinical and experimental studies have shown that the use of phytosterol esters as a food ingredient reduces the plasma concentrations of cholesterol and LDL-cholesterol, not affecting the HDL-cholesterol levels. Many studies have demonstrated the efficacy of these components in a variety of foods, such as margarines. Knowing that there is a strong correlation between artherosclerosis and the plasma LDL levels the use of phytosterols as a food ingredient, can have a beneficial effect on health by reducing the risk of developing artherosclerosis and coronary heart disease. In order to evaluate if milk will be a good food vehicle for phytosterol induce lowering of plasma cholesterol levels we studied 2 groups of 40 Wistar rats each, drinking respectively half-fat and low-fat milk containing phytosterols, during a 30-day feeding period. Milk with different concentrations of phytosterols was used: 0 (as the Control group), 0.2, 0.3, and 0.4 g of phytosterols per 100mL of milk. Throughout the study, clinical observations, body weights and food and milk consumption were measured. The fourth concentrations studied were tolerated as evidenced by the absence of clinical changes in growth, physical behaviour and food and milk habits. The minor changes in hematological parameters were considered to be with no biological or toxicology significance. For the plasma cholesterol concentration there were no significant differences in the cholesterol and HDL levels, in both groups of Wistar rats drinking, either low or half-fat milk. There was a decrease of about 74% (0.2g/100mL) in the LDL levels, with low-fat milk and of about 67% (0.2g/100mL) with half-fat milk. Phytosterols when added to milk did not loose its cholesterol plasma concentration lowering ability.

POP 10

STUDY OF NITRIC OXIDE MOBILIZATION AFTER ERYTHROCYTES STIMULATION WITH ACETYLCHOLINE ON HEALTHY AND SICK PERSONS

F.A. Carvalho, D. Soares, A.V. Maria[1], J. Guerra, M. Martins Prata, L. Caeiro[2], J. Martins-Silva, C. Saldanha
Instituto de Bioquímica, Faculdade de Medicina de Lisboa. Unidade de Biopatologia Vascular, IMM, 1649-028 Lisboa, Portugal.

The nitric oxide (NO) is an important vasodilator messenger interfering in a number of physiological and pathophysiological processes. In this study we stimulated human erythrocytes obtained from patients with different types of diseases (hypercholesterolemia, drepanocytosis, delirium and renal transplantation) with acetylcholine (ACh) and measured the NO production, comparing with the NO levels achieved on erythrocytes of healthy persons. We used human erythrocyte suspensions in sodium chloride 0.9% pH 7 (hematocrit 0.05%) to measure the NO production with a amperometric NO sensor during stimulation with ACh 10 μM. The erythrocytes NO levels, according to the different studied groups, were of 2.8 ± 0.8 nM (delirium; $P<0.001$, n=67), 2.5 ± 0.7 nM (hypercholesterolemia; $P=0.018$, n=17), 5.4 ± 0.8 nM (drepanocytosis; $P<0.001$, n=5) and 2.4 ± 1.2 nM (renal transplantation; n=15) against the 2.0 ± 0.8 nM (n=43) for the control values. We observed the most significant change on the NO production with drepanocytosis erythrocytes samples which could be a positive factor for the compromised tissue oxigenation in this kind of anemia. In conclusion, human erythrocytes of different diseases have different physiological responses to ACh stimulation that leads to changes on NO mobilization mechanisms. The different erythrocytes NO values obtained after ACh stimulation, suggested a future target for vasodilate therapeutic action on a microcirculatory network damaged by different sorts of stimulus.

POS 1

REOXYGENATION AFTER HYPOXIA AND GLUCOSE DEPLETION CAUSES REACTIVE OXYGEN SPECIES PRODUCTION BY MITOCHONDRIA IN HUMAN UMBILICAL VEIN ENDOTHELIAL CELLS (HUVEC).

S Therade-Matharan, E Laemmel, J Duranteau, E Vicaut
Laboratoire d'Etude de la Microcirculation, 10 avenue de Verdun, Faculté de medecine Lariboisière, 75010 Paris, France, Université Paris 7, France

In haemorrhagic shock, local hypoxia is present and followed by reoxygenation during the therapeutic process. In endothelium, reactive oxygen species (ROS) have been identified as a cause of inflammatory reactions and tissular lesions in ischemic territory during reoxygenation. This study was designed to identify the enzymatic mechanisms of ROS formation during reoxygenation after hypoxia. As severe shock, *in vivo*, can affect both O_2 and nutriments, we combined hypoxia at a level close to that found in terminal vessels during shock, with glucose depletion, which induces a relevant additional stress. HUVEC underwent 2 hours of hypoxia (pO2~20mmHg) without glucose and one hour of reoxygenation (pO2~120mmHg) with glucose. ROS production was measured by the fluorescent marker 2',7'-dichloro-dihydrofluorescein diacetate, and cell death, by propidium iodide. After one hour of reoxygenation, fluorescence had risen by 143% ±17%. Cell death was equal to 8.6% ±2.4% Antimycin A, and stigmatellin, which inhibits the type III mitochondrial respiratory chain complex, reduced ROS production to values of 61% ±10% and 59% ±7% respectively, but inhibitors of other chain complexes did not affect it. Neither was the increase in fluorescence affected by inhibition of NADPH oxidase, xanthine oxidase, NO synthase, cyclo-oxygenase, cytochrome p450 monooxygenase, or monoamine oxidase. We did not observe any increase in cell death. These results show that in HUVEC, mitochondria are responsible for ROS production after hypoxia and reoxygenation, and suggest that a ROS release site is activated in the cytochrome b of the type III respiratory chain complex.

POS 2

THE DIASTOLIC FUNCTION OF LEFT VENTRICLE IN HYPERTENSIVE PATIENTS WITH DIABETES MELLITUS TYPE II

C.Tudorica, M.Moise*, M.Muraru,D.Spataru, S.Tudorica**,I.Bruckner
Cardiology Department, Coltea Hospital; * Diagnostic and Treatment Center Dr.Victor Babes; **Ambulatory Masina de Paine, Bucharest, Romania

The aim of the study was to evaluate the diastolic function of left ventricle in patients with systemic hypertension (SH) and diabetes mellitus type II (DM II) that had a normal systolic function of left ventricle(LV). Material and methods: we have studied 110 patients with stable systemic hypertension, M/F ratio 7/4, age between 54 and 72 years (medium age 56,5 years), from whom 52 patients with DM II (more than 3 years diagnosticated) - the study group, and 58 patients without DM II - the control group.Like methods we used clinical examination; standard ECG ; transthoracic echocardiography M, 2 D, Doppler (for evaluation of ejection fraction - EF, E wave peak velocity/ A wave peak velocity - E/A, isovolumic relaxation time - IVRT, left ventricular mass - LV mass). Exclusion criteria: valvulopaties, cardiomiopathies, pericardities, heart failure. All the patients had a normal systolic function (EF > 60%). The results after the evaluation of echocardiographic parameters of diastolic function of left ventricle correlated with LV mass average were: in the study group at LV mass 117,6 g/m^2 - 6 pts had normal diastolic function of LV and 14 altered one, at 147,7 g/m^2- 5 pts had normal diastolic function of LV and 27 altered one;in the control group at LV mass 106,4 g/m^2- 16 pts had normal diastolic function of LV and 12 modified one, at 147,4 g/m^2- 8 pts had normal diastolic function of LV and 16 altered one. Conclusions: the diastolic function is strongly influenced by the presence of diabetes mellitus. It also is related to the presence of the ventricular hypertrophy.

POS 3

COMBINATION OF MENADIONE AND VEGF RELIEVES THEIR INDIVIDUAL EFFECTS ON THE PARACELLULAR PERMEABILITY OF A BRAIN ENDOTHELIAL CELL MONOLAYER INDEPENDENTLY OF P38.

K. Voigt, K. Hartmann, J. Kraus, M. Clauss
Department of Neurology, University Hospital Giessen, D-35385 Giessen, Germany; MPI for Physiological and Clinical Research, D-61231 Bad Nauheim, Germany

Objective: Menadione can cross the lipid bilayer and is therefore considered as an intracellular oxyradical producing agent. VEGF has been reported to induce endothelial permeability, possibly via p38. We examined whether exposure of a monolayer of cultured brain endothelial cells to both agents increases blood-brain barrier permeability in vitro. Methods: The immortalized endothelioma cell line bEnd5 from mouse brain capillaries was grown to confluence on semipermeable filters, and we determined the paracellular permeability of radioactive [^{14}C]-sucrose and [^{3}H]-inulin across the endothelioma monolayers after exposure to 300μM menadione during the assay period, or to 40ng/ml VEGF for 3 hours before the assay, or to both. In addition, the experiments were repeated after preincubation for 30 minutes with the p38-inhibitor SB202190. Results: Exposure to menadione or VEGF alone increased the permeability of the bEnd5 cells significantly; this was less pronounced for menadione than VEGF. Combination of VEGF and menadione still lead to a significant increase of permeability as compared to unstimulated controls, but significantly attenuated their individual effects. The results were the same after inhibition of p38. Conclusion: The results show that the combination of menadione, as a generator of intracellular oxidative stress, and VEGF relieves their individual permeabilizing effects in the mouse brain endothelial cell line bEnd5 independently of p38. Therefore, intracellular free radicals and VEGF may have interactive effects upstream of p38.

POS 4

COMBINATION OF THE PERMEABILIZING EFFECTS OF HYDROGEN PEROXIDE AND VEGF ATTENUATES BRAIN ENDOTHELIAL PERMEABILITY IN VITRO INDEPENDENTLY OF P38.

K. Voigt, K. Hartmann, J. Kraus, M. Clauss
Department of Neurology, University Hospital Giessen, D-35385 Giessen, Germany; MPI for Physiological and Clinical Research, D-61231 Bad Nauheim, Germany

Objective: Free radicals such as hydrogen peroxide can impair blood-brain barrier function. VEGF has been reported to induce endothelial permeability, possibly via p38. We studied whether exposure of a monolayer of cultured brain endothelial cells to both agents increases endothelial permeability in vitro. Methods: The immortalized endothelioma cell line bEnd5 from mouse brain capillaries was grown to confluence on semipermeable filters, and the paracellular permeability of radioactive [^{14}C]-sucrose and [^{3}H]-inulin across the endothelioma monolayers was determined after exposure to 500μM hydrogen peroxide during the assay period, or to 40ng/ml VEGF for 3 hours before the assay, or to both. Additionally, the experiments were repeated after preincubation for 30 minutes with the p38-inhibitor SB202190. Results: Exposure to hydrogen peroxide or VEGF alone lead to a significant increase of the permeability of the bEnd5 cells; this was even more pronounced for hydrogen peroxide than VEGF. Combination of hydrogen peroxide and VEGF still significantly increased permeability as compared to unstimulated controls, but their individual effects were significantly relieved. Inhibition of p38 did not influence the results. Conclusion: The results show that the combination of hydrogen peroxide and VEGF attenuates their individual permeabilizing effects in the mouse brain endothelial cell line bEnd5 independently of p38. Thus, oxidative stress and VEGF may have interactive effects upstream of p38.

POS 5

INCREASED OXIDATIVE STRESS IN MESENTERIC ARTERY FROM HYPERTENSIVE RATS WITH ACTIVATION OF THE RENIN-ANGIOTENSIN SYSTEM

T. Sousa[1], M. Morato[1,4], D. Pinho[1], E. Fernandes[2], F. Carvalho[3], A. Albino-Teixeira[1]
[1]Institute of Pharmacology and Therapeutics, Faculty of Medicine of Porto; [2]REQUIMTE/Physical Chemistry Department, [3]REQUIMTE, Toxicology Department, [4]Pharmacology Department, Faculty of Pharmacy of Porto. University of Porto, Portugal.

Treatment of rats with the adenosine antagonist 1,3-dipropyl-8-sulfophenylxanthine (DPSPX) causes a hypertensive state which is accompanied by vascular hyperplasia and hypertrophy and increased plasma levels of renin activity and angiotensin II (Ang II). Since Ang II stimulates the generation of reactive oxygen species (ROS), we aimed at evaluating the mesenteric artery activity of NADPH oxidase, and glutathione peroxidase (GPx) in DPSPX-induced hypertension. Sham and DPSPX(90 μg/kg/h, i.p., 7 days)-treated rats were used. Systolic blood pressure (SBP) was measured by the tail cuff method. Rats were sacrificed on day 14. NADPH oxidase activity was evaluated by the NBT reduction assay. GPx activity was evaluated by following NADPH oxidation. DPSPX increased SBP (day 14: 142.6Γ3.4* vs 115.0Γ2.2; mmHg, * p<0.05 vs sham, n=11). NADPH oxidase and GPx activities were increased in hypertensive rats when compared to sham (NADPH oxid: 254.8Γ57.5* vs 100.0Γ14.4, n=9; GPx: 132.0Γ4.0* vs 100.0Γ4.5, n=6; meanΓS.E.M.; results are as % of sham activity; *p<0.05 vs sham).

We can conclude that this hypertension is associated with increased mesenteric artery generation of ROS by NADPH oxidase, which is accompanied by an increase of the antioxidant activity of GPx.

Saturday, 11th September
Poster Presentation – Smooth Muscle Cell Biology (PSM)

PSM 1

THE EFFECTS OF R-CADHERIN/CATENIN ON SMOOTH MUSCLE CELLS PROLIFERATION OF PULMONARY ARTERY ARE ASSOCIATED WITH HYPOXIC PULMONARY HYPERTENSION.

Wenjun LI, Huifeng YU, Xucheng JIANG and Fengmei Chen
Department of Pathology, Shanghai Second Medical University, 200025, Shanghai, China.

Objectives: cadherin/catenin complex is crucial to cell-cell adhesion and proliferation. Smooth muscle cells (SMCs) proliferation is an important step of pulmonary vascular structure remodeling (PVSR) in hypoxic pulmonary hypertension (HPH), but the mechanism is less well understood. Thus, we hypothesized that R-cadherin/catenin may play a critical role on PVSR in HPH. *Methods and Results:* We examined the expression of R-cadherin, β-catenin, cyclinD1 and c-myc in SMCs of pulmonary artery in rat with HPH in vivo and in primary cultured SMCs treated with hypoxic conditioned medium in vitro by immunohistochemistry. Compared with control, the expression of R-cadherins and membrane β-catenin are significantly reduced both in vitro and in vivo (all P<0.01). These changes of R-cadherin and membrane β-catenin coincided with the detection of nuclear β-catenin and elevated cyclinD1 expression (both P<0.05). But no significant change of c-myc expression was observed (both P>0.05). Furthermore, R-cadherin neutralizing antibodies remarkably increased the amount of nuclear β-catenin, the expression of cyclinD1 and the proliferation of SMCs cultured with hypoxic conditioned medium (P<0.01, P<0.01 and P<0.05 respectively). Tyrosine kinase inhibitor tyrphostine 25, however, reduced the expression of nuclear β-catenin and cyclinD1 and inhibited proliferation of SMCs cultured with hypoxic conditioned medium (all P<0.05). *Conclusions:* Down-regulation of E-cadherin expression and tyrosine phosphorylation of β-catenin lead to accumulation of nuclear β-catenin, which results in SMCs proliferation in HPH via cell cycle start.

PTO 1

IMPROVEMENT IN MICROCIRCULATORY PARAMETERS AFTER REPEATED SHORT-TERM PGE-1 THERAPY IN AUTOIMMUNE DISORDERS

Z.Pencz,V.Kristóf",Á.Laczkó",É.Weinberger,E.Szakály,E.Varga,A.Sásdi
2nd Department of Internal Medicine,Péterfy Hospital,1074 Budapest, Hungary
"Clinic of Cardiovascular Surgery,Semmelweis University,1124 Budapest, Hungary

Autoimmune disorders involve about 0,5-1% of the population in Middle Europe.These diseases often cause Raynaud's phenomenon /RP/, microangiopathy, hardly curable ulcers and gangrene of the extremities.

The aim of this poster was to evaluate the efficacy of repeated /6 week intervals short-term alprostadil therapy and to measure microcirculatory changes. Besides the conventional, basic therapy 14 previously selected for responder state patients were treated with PGE1. Nine of them suffered from progressive systemic sclerosis, three of them from rheumatoid arthri-tis and two of them from systemic lupus erythematosus. None of them had got significant macroangiopathy.All patients had got ulcers on the extremi- ties and suffered from severe RP.They received 3 hour infusions of alprostadil 40-60ug/day–depends on tolerability on 5 consecutive days. Before and after 5 days therapy transcutan O2 pressure measurement and capillaroscopy were performed. Healing of acral lesions, severity of pain, number and severity of RP attacks were also evaluated. The treatments increased the tcpO2 values 31%, 34%, 30%, 36% and the number of existing nailfold capillaries 15%, 21%, 24%, 26% and reduced the frequency of RP symptoms 36%, 42%, 46%, 44% and the severity of pain 32%, 41%, 35%, 45% visual analog scale from baseline after the first, second, third and fourth periods, respectively.

Our study suggests that repeated, short–term PGE1 therapy is effective, the microcirculatory changes are significant. The hospitalisation is short and the costs are relatively low.

PTO 2

EFFECT OF DIETARY SUPPLEMENTATION WITH ISOSORBIDE 5-MONONITRATE ON VASCULAR/PLATELET CONSTRICTOR BALANCE IN CYCLOSPORIN-A INDUCED HYPERTENSIVE RATS

F. Reis, L. Ponte, L. Almeida, T. Alcobia, C. Costa-Almeida, F. Teixeira.
Institute of Pharmacology and Experimental Therapeutics, Medicine Faculty, Coimbra University, 3004-504 Coimbra, Portugal

To assess the effect of an organic NO donor (Isosorbide 5-Mononitrate: Is-5-Mn) treatment on prevention and/or regression of Cyclosporin A (CsA)-induced hypertension and on NO-cGMP pathway, TXA_2/PGI_2 balance and peripheral 5-HT contents. Five rat groups were tested: control, CsA (5 mg/kg/day) and Is-5-Mn (150 mg/kg/day, bid) groups were treated for 7 wks; preventive Is-5-Mn group: Is-5-Mn for 2 wks plus Is-5-Mn+CsA for 7 wks (Is-5-Mn+CsA); regressive Is-5-Mn group: CsA for 7 wks plus CsA+Is-5-Mn for 5 wks (CsA+Is-5-Mn). Results are means ± SEM (ANOVA/Fisher's: *P<0.05,**P<0.01,***P<0.001 vs CsA). CsA-induced SBP and DBP increase was prevented, but not reverted, by concomitant Is-5-Mn treatment. In the Is-5-Mn+CsA group, the CsA-evoked vascular/ platelet NOS activity ([^{3}H]-citrulline formation) and cGMP contents (immunoassay) disturbances were prevented; AA-evoked TXA_2/PGI_2 balance (immunoassays) was unaffected and plasma 5-HT (HPLC-ED) was even reduced vs CsA. In the CsA+Is-5-Mn group, NO-cGMP impairment was maintained, while TXA_2/PGI_2 ratio (0.034±0.011**) was even higher and plasma and platelet 5-HT (2.6±0.6 ng/ml; 1715±115 pg/10^9plat.***) were maintained vs the CsA group (0.006±0.001; 3.0±0.5 ng/ml; 629±46 pg/10^9plat.). In conclusion, Is-5-Mn treatment prevented CsA-induced hypertension and the underlying NO-cGMP disturbances without negative effects on TXA_2/PGI_2 balance and 5-HT levels. In opposition, when tested after CsA, no reversion of hypertension occurred, while the constrictor balance even worsened, recommending a judicious evaluation of the nitrate therapy impact in order to avoid further cardiovascular side effects.

PTV 1

MODULATION OF HUMAN COLON CARCINOMA CELL INVASIVENESS BY DOWNREGULATION OF b1 INTEGRINS.

J. Niewiarowska, M. Wiktorska, I. Papiewska, I. Sacewicz, M. Ugorski, A. Okruszek, C.S. Cierniewski
Department of Molecular and Medical Biophysics, Medical University in Lodz, 92-215 Lodz, Poland

As with many types of cancer, cell motility is an important factor in the progression and metastasis of colon cancers. The purpose of this study was to delineate the role of adhesive receptors in migration of various colon carcinoma cell lines differing in invasiveness, and to identify specific targets to prevent their motility. These cells significantly differed in the extracellular signal-regulated kinase $(ERK)^{MAPK}/p38^{SAPK}$ activity ratio, and thus were predicted to have various ability to proliferate or to enter the state of dormancy *in vivo*. To evaluate invasiveness of cancer cells, we analyzed their chemotactic migration across the ECM-coated membrane. Their adhesive properties were also characterized by the analysis of both adhesion and migration to fibronectin, laminin and collagen. In addition, the expression of major integrin subunits, the selected intact β1 integrins, and other adhesive receptors (ICAM, E-selectin, uPAR) was analyzed by flow cytometry. Invasiveness of these cells was strongly correlated with the expression of β1 integrin subunit, and, to a lesser extent, with uPAR. Inhibition of β1 integrin subunit by DNAzyme to β1 mRNA significantly decreased chemotactic migration. Inhibition of β1 integrin expression almost abolished invasiveness of the cells that showed high activity of $(ERK)^{MAPK}$ and undetectable activity $p38^{SAPK}$ (HT29, SW620, LS180, LOVO). Invasiveness of carcinoma cells with low $(ERK)^{MAPK}$ and high $p38^{SAPK}$ activity was much less affected (CX1/1, CX1/1Q8). These data showed that downregulation of β1 integrin subunit is sufficient to inhibit invasiveness and migration of some, but not all colon carcinoma cells.

PTV 2

VASCULAR MATURATION IN THE TUMOUR AND ITS ROLE IN DETERMINING RESPONSE TO TUBULIN-BINDING VASCULAR TARGETING AGENTS

C.R. Ireson, S.A. Hill, G. Lewis, V. Prise, A. Steele, C. Coralli, G.U. Dachs, P.R. Barber, D. Honess, C. Kanthou, D. Shima[1] and G. Tozer
Gray Cancer Institute, Mount Vernon Hospital, Northwood, HA6 2JR
[1]Eyetech Research Center, Woburn, MA019801, USA

Combretastatin A-4-phosphate (CA-4-P), the lead tubulin-binding vascular targeting agent, shuts down blood flow in many human tumour xenografts. Although the specific tumour characteristics determining susceptibility to CA-4-P have not been established, it may be a consequence of an immature vasculature with relatively little smooth muscle actin (SMA). Fibrosarcoma cell lines, which express only single VEGF isoforms, were developed from corresponding knock-out mice and grown s.c. in SCID mice. Tumours were excised, stained for SMA & CD-31 and % of SMA-stained vessels calculated (vascular maturity index). VMI was 30, 70 & 100% for $VEGF_{120}$, w/t & $VEGF_{188}$ tumours respectively, confirming the role of the high molecular weight isoform in vascular maturation. Tumours were also grown in dorsal skin flap window chambers in SCID mice for intravital microscopy. Fragments of $VEGF_{120}$ tumours expanded rapidly in the chambers despite poor internal vascularization. Within 4 days of implantation, haemorrhage of the surrounding blood vessels was observed. In contrast, $VEGF_{188}$ tumours had a relatively organised vasculature, with narrower vessels and no haemorrhage. Red blood cell velocity was 25 and 100% of pre-treatment values in $VEGF_{120}$ and $VEGF_{188}$ tumours respectively, 24h following administration of a single i.v. dose of CA-4-P (30 mg/kg). These data suggest that morphological and functional characteristics impinge on the responsiveness of tumour blood vessels to vascular targeting agents.
This work was supported by Cancer Research UK.

PTV 3

FAILING ANGIOADAPTATION IN TUMOR MICROCIRCULATION

Annemiek J.M. Cornelissen[1], Beata Styp-Rekowska[1], Anouk A. Sloot[1,2], Timothy W. Secomb[4], Martin Eichhorn[3], Axel R. Pries[1]
[1]Dept. of Physiology, Charité University Medicine, Berlin, Arnimallee 22 14195 Berlin, Germany; [2]TUDelft, the Netherlands; [3]Ludwig Maximilians University, Munich, Germany; [4]University of Arizona, Tuscon, USA

In comparison to normal healthy microvasculature the architecture of tumor microcirculation exhibits a high degree of structural and functional heterogeneity. Here we test whether changes in reaction of microvessels to angioadaptive stimuli might explain the observed discrepancies.

Intravital microscopy was used to record microvascular networks in the rat mesentery and an A-Mel-3 tumor. The topology, diameter, length, and red blood cell velocity were measured. A previously validated model simulation was used to estimate pressure (P), flow (Q), and shear stress (τ). The adaptation of vessel diameters in response to hemodynamic (P,Q), metabolic (pO_2), and conducted stimuli was predicted. Adaptation characteristics optimized for normal microvascular beds (standard) were compared with characteristics changed to simulate tumor conditions ('tumor': reduced hemodynamic sensitivity, reduced information transfer and randomized metabolic sensitivity). To quantify the functional network properties, the variation of τ (τ_{var}) at branch points was calculated.

For the experimental measured diameters (no adaptation) τ_{var} in the mesentery network was low in comparison to the tumor network (2.07 vs. 9.66). For both networks, τ_{var} was low (1.32 and 0.88) after simulated adaptation with standard parameters and high (8.21 and 10.02) after adaptation with 'tumor' parameters. In conclusion: These data show that typical functional properties of tumor microvascular networks may be explained by specific changes in the assumed adaptation responses of vessel diameter irrespective of network topology.

PVF 1

THE ASSESSMENT OF MICROALBUMINURIA IN DIABETIC AND HYPERTENSIVE PATIENTS AFTER TREATMENT WITH CARVEDILOLUM AND TELMISARTAN

C.Tudorica, M.Moise*, S.Tudorica**, M.Muraru, D.Spataru, I.Bruckner
Cardiology Department, Coltea Hospital; * Diagnostic and Treatment Center Dr.Victor Babes; **Ambulatory Masina de Paine, Bucharest, Romania

The aim of the study was to observe the influence of carvedilolum and telmisartan on albuminuria in diabetic and hypertensive patients and also on the left ventricular end diastolic diameter-LVEDD and the ejection fraction-EF Material:we have studied 81 patients with diabetes mellitus type II known about 3,5 years and stable systemic hypertension, M/F ratio: 35/46, medium age 60,7 years.All of them were hospitalized. When they left the hospital they were diagnosticated with NYHA I, II or III heart failure, 40 of them were treated with diuretics, carvedilolum (up to 37,5 mg/day) and telmisartan (80 mg/day)-A group; 41 of them were on diuretics, carvedilolum (the same doses) and perindoprilum (4 mg/day) or enalaprilum (40 mg/day)-B group. Method: albuminuria 24 hours, standard ECG, transthoracic echocardiography M and 2D Mode (for LVEDD, EF) at the beginning of the treatment and at 3, 6 and 12 months. Results: in the A group albuminuria decreased from 275,4 to 156,2 g/24 hours, EF raised from 48,7% to 43,2%, LVEDD decreased from 62,3 to 56,2 mm.In B group albuminuria decreased from 272,6 to 180,5 g/24 hours, EF raised from 42,8% to 45,9% and LVEDD was reduced from 62,5 to 58,1 mm. Conclusion: In both groups we can observe a decrease of albuminuria 24 hours (consecutively to an improvement of renal microcirculation), more important in those patients treated with telmisartan.The benefic effect on left ventricular end diastolic diameter and ejection fraction it is possible to be the consequence of a better left ventricular walls microcirculation (none of these patients associated revascularisation tehniques).

PVF 2

ACETYLCHOLINESTERASE (AChE), A NEW MARKER OF CHRONIC VENOUS DISEASES

Pereira Albino, Carlota Saldanha, Martins e Silva
Instituto de Bioquimica da F.M.L, Lisboa, Portugal
Unidade de A. e Cirurgia Vascular H. Pulido Valente, Lisboa, Portugal

It is consensual that venous hypertension cause leucocyte sequestration in the microcirculation. The leucocytes adhere to the endothelium of the post capillary venule and promote an inflamatory reaction. This reaction is systemic and has been detected in patients with venous diseases where upper limbs showed more leucocytes sequestration than the control subjects. However it is not exactly proved, in vivo, the leucocyte endothelium interaction. The extra-neuronal localisation of the acethylcholinesterase (AChE) in leucocyte and venules endothelium supported the hypothesis of this protein have other function besides the catalyte one. In Previsious works, we found an increase in AChE activity in patients with essential hypertension, and also the inibition of AChE induces an inverse of leucocyte-endothelium interaction by inversing cAMP dependent cytokines (IL-1B) release to blood circulation. This supports that AChE can be a mediator of leucocyte endothelium interaction.
Aim of the study: to verify the enzyme activity of erithrocitary AChE in patients with confirm chronic venous diseases. AChE was determined in venous whole blood samples collected from the forearm of the patients and the results were compared with a normal population.
Methods: 65 patients with chronic venous diseases (C2 to C5) (mean age: 46 years) was analysed to determine, in conjuntion with other hemorreologic parameters (hematocrit, leucocytes,whole viscosity, fibrinogen, erythrocyte aggregation), the AChE, by Ellman´s spectrophotometric method modified by Kaplan.
Results: In all the patients, with documented venous hypertension, has been detected a significant elevation of the AChE (normal 160-257 mean 250 UI/min/mgHb; patients 234-415 mean 306.82UI (min/mgHb).
Conclusion: Increase in the erithrocitary AChE activity is related with leucocyte activity and can confirm the existence of a leucocyte-endothelium interaction in patients with venous hypertension, it can be used as a marker of chronic venous diseases

OAT 1

ESTIMATION OF O_2 CONSUMPTION RATE OF ARTERIOLAR WALLS IN SKELETAL MUSCLE

M. Shibata, S. Ichioka, J. Ando, A. Kamiya
Department of Biomedical Engineering, University of Tokyo
- Tokyo 113-0033, Japan

Recent studies suggest the possibility of O_2 supply from arterioles to surrounding tissue, since a significant drop of O_2 levels in the arterioles was demonstrated. However, the magnitude of the drop in pO_2 in arterioles is too large to be explained by diffusion alone. In this study, we evaluated the involvement of O_2 consumption by arteriolar walls in the pO_2 drop in arterioles of skeletal muscle under physiological conditions.
To estimate the O_2 consumption rate of arteriolar walls we measured the intra and perivascular pO_2 of arterioles in rat cremaster muscle, both at resting and vasodilating states by phosphorescence quenching technique. Using measured pO_2 gradients across the arteriolar walls, O_2 consumption rates of both conditions were determined based on Krogh-Erlang analysis.
We found a significant drop in pO_2 in the arterioles after branching and the presence of a large pO_2 gradient across the arteriolar wall. The O_2 consumption rates in the arteriolar walls estimated from the pO_2 values ranged from 1.8×10^{-2} ml/s/g (large arterioles) to 0.8×10^{-2} ml/s/g (small arterioles) at rest, and from 0.9×10^{-2} (large) to 0.7×10^{-2} ml/s/g (small) when dilated. These values are 10-100 times higher than the values of vascular segments or vascular cell suspensions measured by in vitro experiments. These findings not only support the hypothesis that O_2 can be supplied from arterioles, but also suggest arterioles play more important role in distributing the blood supply to other organs by restricting blood inflow to skeletal muscle under resting condition even if a large amount of O_2 is consumed by the vessel walls themselves.

OAT 2

A NEW MODEL FOR *in vivo* EVALUATION OF MICROVASCULAR REACTIVTY IN MAN. THE EFFECTS OF ANGIOTENSIN II.

A.J.H.M. Houben, J.P. Burgwinkel, P.W. de Leeuw.
Dept. of Int. Medicine, University Hospital Maastricht, CARIM, PO Box 5800, 6202 AZ Maastricht, The Netherlands.

The aim of the present study was to develop a new model to study directly in vivo human microcirculatory reactivity to the effects of locally applied drugs. Since Ang II is highly relevant in cardiovascular regulating proces-ses, the effects of this hormone were studied in particular. Design and me-thods: 31 (18F/13M) normotensive subjects were studied (mean age 21 ± 2 (SD) years). Bulbar conjunctival arterioles and venules were recorded using intravital microscopy, before and after application of placebo eye-drops in one eye, and Ang II (0.01%), or phenylephrine (0.25%) drops in the other eye (in random order). Microvascular diameter changes were measured using dedicated software. Results: Repeated analyses of the same microvessels (n=5 subjects) revealed a variability of measurement of 4%. The repeated measurements of microvascular diameters following placebo eye-drops resulted in a variability of arteriolar diameters of 2%, and 4% for venular diameters. Ang II induced a median arteriolar constriction of 20% (11-20 interq.range) ($p<0.01$ vs placebo) and a median venular constriction of 13% (5-16) ($p<0.01$ vs placebo). As a positive control phenylephrine drops were applied, which induced an arteriolar constriction of 15% (11-21) ($p<0.01$ vs placebo), and a venular constriction of 16% (10-26) ($p<0.05$ vs placebo). This constriction of both drugs lasted for at least 10 minutes. Conclusions: We present a new model for in vivo testing of microvascular reactivity to locally applied drugs in man with low variability. Angiotensin II acutely induced a constriction of conjunctival arterioles and venules, which lasted for at least 10 minutes. These data suggest that this in vivo model is suitable for studying the renin-angiotensin system in the human microcirculation.

OAT 3

TWO-PHOTON LASER SCANNING MICROSCOPIC IMAGING OF WALL STRUCTURES IN LARGE MOUSE ARTERIES.

R.T.A. Megens[1],W. Engels[1], M.G.A. oude Egbrink[2], D.W. Slaaf[1,3], M.A.M.J. van Zandvoort[1].
Departments of [1]Biophysics; and [2]Physiology, Cardiovascular Research Intstitute Maastricht, University of Maastricht, P.O. Box 616, 6200MD Maastricht, The Netherlands. [3]Department of Biomedical Engineering, Technical University Eindhoven, P.O. box 513, 5600MB, Eindhoven, The Netherlands.

Atherogenesis involves structural and cellular changes in the arterial wall. Imaging of such structures and cells requires optical sectioning and large penetration depth. Two-photon laser scanning microscopy (TPLSM) combines good optical sectioning properties with a large penetration depth, high resolution, and reduced photo damage. In the present study, we use TPLSM to study intact large arteries that are prone to atherogenesis.
We imaged mouse carotid arteries in an ex vivo or in vivo setup. In the ex vivo setup, an isolated artery is mounted in a home built perfusion chamber and imaged using a water dipping objective (40x, NA=0.8 or 60x, NA=1.0). Vessels were studied at a transmural pressure of 80mmHg without flow. In the in vivo setup (same objectives), the anesthetized mouse is positioned on the microscope stage with the carotid artery exposed. To reduce motional disturbances due to heart beat and respiration, a triggering system is used to acquire images at the same stage of the cardiac cycle. This resulted in relatively stable optical sections.
Elastin is visualized using eosin, nuclei (DNA/RNA) are visualized using SYTO13. In both models, the elastin network and cellular components, such as endothelial and smooth muscle cells, are clearly visible.
The use of this new imaging technique with enhanced penetration depth (TPLSM) combined with triggering of the imaging at a certain stage in the cardiac cycle will enable us to study the development of vascular diseases such as atherosclerosis.

OAT 4

USING FIBERED CONFOCAL FLUORESCENCE MICROSCOPY (CELL-VIZIOTM) FOR EXTENDED IMAGING CAPABILITIES IN THE FIELD OF MICROCIRCULATION. COMPLEMENTARITIES WITH INTRAVITAL MICROSCOPY.

Elisabeth Laemmel[1], Magalie Genet[2], Eric Vicaut[1]
[1]Microvascular Research Laboratory. Department of Biophysics. F. Widal Hospital. 200, Rue du Fbg St Denis. 75475 Paris Cedex 10, France
[2]Mauna Kea Technologies. 9, Rue d'Enghien 75010 Paris, France

This study investigated the capability of Fibered Confocal Fluorescence Microscopy (FCFM) to provide in vivo microvascular observations in the context of microvascular research. In the first part of the study, we compared the main characteristics of FCFM with those of Intravital Fluorescence Microscopy (IFM). An intravital mouse cremaster preparation was used as a common basis to allow for imaging with both modalities. We discussed the feasibility of obtaining quantitative measurements usually provided by IFM in the context of FCFM: morphometry, vaso-constriction and dilation effects, as well as red blood cells (RBCs) velocity. Phototoxicity issues were also discussed. In the second part of the study, we investigated complementarities between FCFM and IFM. Limitations of FCFM were also investigated. We shown that the real-time capability of the system, as well as the flexibility and small diameter of the optical probe allow for the exploration of organs with limited accessibility such as kidney, liver, mesentery or conjunctiva. We conclude that FCFM allows performing observations and measurements usually provided by IFM and that the micro-invasiveness of FCFM provides extended imaging capabilities for in vivo in situ observations when compared to IFM.

OAT 6

ARE DIRECT AND INDIRECT CAPILLARY PRESSURE MEASUREMENTS COMPARABLE?

J.C. de Graaff[1], D.Th. Ubbink[2], J.A. van der Spruit[2]2
Dept. of Anaesthesiology[1], St. Antonius Hospital, PO Box 2500, 3430EM Nieuwegein; Dept. of Vascular Surgery[2], Academic Medical Center, Amsterdam, The Netherlands.

Capillary pressure can be estimated by direct cannulation (using a servo-nulling micropressure system) and by indirect measurements (using the venous occlusion method). The venous occlusion method estimates the whole-organ capillary pressure from the inflection point of a venous pressure tracing after sudden occlusion of venous outflow. With the direct method a single capillary in the skin of a digit is cannulated by a micropipette connected to a servo-nulling micropressure system.
Although the indirect method is simpler, its use remains debatable. Therefore, we compared capillary pressure measured using the indirect (lower leg) and direct capillary method (capillary of the skin in the hallux) in the legs of 7 healthy volunteers in the sitting and supine positions.
Paired measurements could be obtained in 7 subjects in the sitting position and 6 subjects in the supine position. Mean direct capillary pressure (42±23 mm Hg) did not differ significantly ($p=0.45$) from the indirect capillary pressure (40 ± 28 mm Hg). The intraclass correlation coefficient was 0.89 ("good"). However, the difference between both methods was dependent of the magnitude of the pressure values (regression line of the difference plot was significant: -0.6, $p= 0.02$).
Direct and indirect capillary pressure measurements are comparable methods for the estimation of capillary pressure. However, there is a pressure related difference between both methods. This difference can be caused by the difference in measurement site (whole lower leg vs. capillary in the skin of the hallux) or the measurement principle.

OAT 7

SIMULTANEOUS MONITORING OF OXYGENATION, BLOOD FLOW, METABOLIC PARAMETERS AND NITRIC OXIDE IN/FROM SMALL AREAS OF THE RAT BRAIN BY VISIBLE SPECTROSCOPY AND LASER DOPPLER.

F.A. Martín*, J.L. Gonzalez-Mora, Mª.L. Luis-García, C. Merino and M.A. Castellano.
Dep. Fisiología. Fac. de Medicina. Univ. de La Laguna, Tenerife, 38007. Islas Canarias. Spain.

The aim of this work was to demonstrate the capabilities of in vivo visible spectroscopy to monitor microcirculation, blood oxygenation and metabolic parameters from small areas of the rat brain jointly with the determination of cerebral blood flow using doppler. Sprague-Dawley rats were anaesthetized for surgical procedure (approved by the local Animal Care and Use Committee). VISChromex was used to obtain and analyze in vivo absorption spectra. Briefly, light from a halogen lamp (100 W) was passed through an optical fiber (100um ϕ) placed in the rat striatum. Scattered light was collected by another optical fiber and sent to a linear CCD detector via a monochromator giving us the possibility of measuring oxyhaemoblobin, deoxyhaemoglobin, nitric oxide, cytochromes b, c and aa3 and even the newly discovered neuroglobin. A laser doppler probe was attached to the optical fibers for simultaneous monitoring of blood flow. It was studied if this approach is sensitive enough for determining the changes induced by different levels of hypoxia or blood flow interruptions by common carotid occlusion. Results show that *in vivo* spectroscopy in combination with doppler is able to detect accurately the changes in microcapillary blood oxygenation, metabolic parameters, nitric oxide and blood flow induced in small areas of the rat brain. In vivo spectroscopy can be used as a very useful tool for gaining insight into the roles of NO, microcirculation and even metabolic parameters in life tissues.

OIR 1

ISCHEMIC PRECONDITIONING IMPROVES THE INTESTINAL OXYGENATION IN REPERFUSION INJURY OF THE INTESTINE

I.H. Mallick, W. Yang, M.C. Winslet, A.M. Seifalian
University Department of Surgery, Royal Free and University College Medical School, London, United Kingdom

Background: Ischemic preconditioning (IPC) provides a way of protecting the intestine from damage inflicted by ischemia reperfusion (IR) injury. This study was designed to evaluate the effect of IPC on the intestinal oxygenation in IR injury.
Methods: Rats were allocated into (a) sham group, (b) IR group consisting of 30 min of intestinal ischemia followed by 2 hr of reperfusion and (c) IPC group, as in IR group, but preceded by 10 min of ischemia and 10 min of reperfusion. Heart rate (HR), arterial oxygen saturation (SaO_2) and mean arterial pressure (MAP) were monitored continuously. Intestinal tissue oxyhemoglobin (HbO_2) and cytochrome oxidase CuA redox state (Cyt Ox) were measured by near infrared reflectance spectroscopy (NIRS). At the end of the reperfusion, blood samples for lactate dehydrogenase (LDH) levels and biopsies of ileum were obtained.
Results: HR and SaO_2 did not change statistically throughout the experiment (p> 0.05). During ischemia there was an increase of MAP from the baseline in both IR (87±3.6 mmHg to 111.5± 4.8 mmHg, p<0.01) and IPC groups (87.7 ±6.5 mm Hg to 111.7±4.6 mm Hg, p < 0.01). IPC improved the HbO_2 and Cyt Ox significantly (p<0.001vs.IR) at the end of the reperfusion. Serum LDH levels were significantly reduced (p<0.001) in IPC (667.1 +/- 86.8) as compared to Group IR (1973.8 +/- 306.5). Histological evaluation demonstrated that IPC reduced the mucosal injury grade (p<0.01 vs. IR).
Conclusion: This study demonstrates that IPC improves the intestinal tissue oxygenation and may be successfully applied during small bowel transplantation.

OIR 2

PLATELET-LEUCOCYTE AND PLATELET-NEUTROPHIL AGGREGATES ARE MARKERS OF THE INFLAMMATORY RESPONSE FOLLOWING INTERMITTENT CLAUDICATION

S Pasupathy, R Young, KM Naseem, S Homer-Vanniasinkam
Vascular Surgical Unit, Leeds General Infirmary, LS1 3EX, UK.

We investigated different platelet markers to identify their utility in demonstrating the inflammatory response observed after intermittent claudication. Methods: Full ethical approval was obtained.14 claudicants and 12 age and sex-matched healthy controls were recruited. All subjects gave consent to exercise on a treadmill until claudication pain (claudicants) or exhaustion (controls). Blood was sampled pre-exercise, immediately post-exercise and 60-minutes post-exercise (recovery) for flow cytometric evaluation of platelet fibrinogen binding, P-selectin expression, platelet-leucocyte aggregation (PLA) and platelet-neutrophil aggregation (PNA). Results are given in medians with statistical analysis using the Wilcoxon signed rank and Mann Whitney U tests. Results: The median age was 65 years. Both cohorts observed an exercise induced rise in platelet fibrinogen binding (claudicants: pre-exercise 0.99% to post-exercise 1.7% p<0.002) and P-selectin expression (claudicants: pre-exercise 0.68% to post-exercise 1.22% p<0.002). After the 60-minute recovery period, these levels had returned to pre-exercise levels in both cohorts. Similarly, PLA and PNA levels rose after exercise in both cohorts (claudicants PLA: pre-exercise 6.7% to post-exercise 9.2% p<0.002; claudicants PNA: pre-exercise 6.8% to post-exercise 9.1% p<0.002). In contrast, after the 60-minute recovery period, PLA and PNA levels remained high only in the claudicant cohort (PLA claudicants 10.4% vs controls 7.1% p=0.009, PNA claudicants 9.9% vs controls 7.0% p=0.004). Conclusions: Platelet fibrinogen binding and P-selectin expression are transiently increased after exercise in both claudicants and controls. However PLA and PNA levels are persistently increased after exercise only in claudicants.

OIR 3

INHIBITION OF RHO KINASE IMPROVES VASCULAR ENOS FUNCTION DURING RENAL ISCHEMIA REPERFUSION

A.M.G. Versteilen, R.J.P Musters, A.B.J Groeneveld, I. Korstjens, P. SipkemaDepartment of Physiology, Institute for Cardiovascular Research, VUUniversity medical center, 1081 BT Amsterdam, The Netherlands

Renal ischemia reperfusion (I/R) results in an altered renal vasoreactivity and impaired organ blood flow. This results in a reduction of oxygen delivery to the renal tubular tissue leading to apoptotic cell death and organ failure. We investigated the effect of the Rho kinase inhibitor Y27632 on renal blood flow, vasoreactivity, F-actin and eNOS in I/R. Male Wistar rats were subjected to 60 minutes bilateral clamping of the renal arteries. The group treated with the Rho kinase inhibitor received one hour before clamping 1 mg/kg Y27632 or sham. After clamping the kidneys were reperfused for one hour. Renal blood flow was measured with fluorescent microspheres. The impaired blood flow (3.04±0.35 ml/min/g) after I/R was prevented by the Rho kinase inhibitor (5.37±0.52, ml/min/g, P<0.05). Renal vascular reactivity to norepinephrine and acetylcholine was measured in a pressure myograph. The NO mediated acetylcholine response, which was nearly absent after I/R was preserved by the Rho kinase inhibitor. Vascular endothelial F-actin morphology and eNOS localization was visualized by fluorescent 3D digital imaging microscopy. The formation of endothelial F-actin fibers and loss of perinuclear localization of eNOS, which is associated with a loss of function was prevented by the Rho kinase inhibitor after I/R. These findings indicate that inhibition of Rho kinase preserves renal blood flow and vascular eNOS function probably by modulation of the F-actin cytoskeleton.

OIR 4

THE EFFECTS OF MELATONIN ON ISCHEMIA REPERFUSION INJURY IN RAT PIAL MICROCIRCULATION

D. Lapi, F. Vetri, P.L. Marchiafava,A.Colantuoni*
*Department of Neuroscience, "Federico II" University Medical School, 80131 Naples, and Department of Physiology and Biochemistry, 56127 Pisa, Italy

The aim of the present study was to assess the effects of melatonin on microvascular changes induced by ischemia reperfusion injury in rat pial microcirculation. The study was approved by the local University ethical Committee. Pial microcirculation of male Wistar rats was visualized by fluorescence microscopy through an open cranial window, using fluorescein isothiocyanate bound to dextran (MW 70 kD) as a tracer. Vessel diameter, permeability increase, number of leukocytes adhering to venular walls and capillary red blood cell velocity were determined by computer-assisted methods. Melatonin (0.5 -1- 2 mg/kg body wt., i.v.) was administered 10 min before bilateral occlusion of carotid artery for 30 min, and at the start of reperfusion lasting 60 min. In control animals, ischemia caused constriction of arterioles (-20 ± 4% of baseline, order 4); reperfusion induced differentiated responses: constriction within 40 min (-20 ± 3%). Moreover, there were increase in permeability (0.45 ± 0.05 Normalized Grey Levels) and adhesion of leukocytes (8 ± 2/100 mm venular length). Melatonin caused dose-dependent responses: at the highest dosage, arteriolar dilation within 40 min of reperfusion (+ 18 ± 3%). Moreover, permeability increase (0.15 ± 0.03 NGL) and adhesion of leukocytes (2 ± 1/100 μm venular length) (p<0.01 vs. control) were prevented. Capillary red blood cell velocity increased compared with control (0.32 ± 0.03 vs. 0.24 ± 0.02 mm/s). In conclusion, melatonin protected cerebral capillary perfusion and reduced damage in blood-brain barrier function.

OIR 5

THE EFFECT OF ISCHAEMIC PRECONDITIONING ON TISSUE OXYGENATION AND MITOCHONDRIA FUNCTION OF THE FATTY LIVER

W. Yang, G. Glanzunious, P. Wignarajah, J-W. Taanman, M.C.Winslet, A.M. Seifalian
University Department of Surgery, Royal Free and University College Medical School, London, United Kingdom

Background: Fatty liver are used as marginal donors in liver transplantation. Very little is known about the mechanisms of ischaemia reperfusion injury (IRI). This study was aimed to establish whether cytochrome oxidase c (CytOx) activity is compromised by ischaemia reperfusion injury in fatty liver and whether ischaemic preconditioning (IPC) can protect liver from IRI through improving CytOx activity. **Methods:** New Zealand rabbits (3-3.5kg) were fed on a high cholesterol diet for 8 weeks to induce moderate hepatic steatosis. Animals were then allocated to three groups: Ischaemic group (IR, n=6), underwent 60 min lobe ischaemia followed by 7 hrs of reperfusion; Ischemic preconditioning group (IPC, n=8), subjected to 5 min ischaemia and 10 min ischaemia and then 60 min ischaemia followed by 7 hrs of reperfusion; control group (Sham,n=6) underwent same surgical procedure but no ischaemia was induced. Hepatic tissue CytOx radix status was continuously monitored in vivo by near infrared spectroscopy (NIRS) and liver tissue biopsies were collected at baseline, 2 and 7 hrs of reperfusion for the measurement of CytOx and citrate syntheses activities in vitro. **Results:** IR group had reduced CytOx radix status *in vivo* and CytOx activity measured *in vitro*. IPC group showed higher levels CytOx status at the end of 7 hrs of reperfusion as compared with IR group ($p<0.01$) and that was in line with well preserved CytOx activity ($p<0.05$). **Conclusion:** This study suggests that IPC reduces IRI in fatty livers by improving CytOx activity. CytOx radox status monitored in vivo correlates well with CytOx activity.

OIR 6

THE ENDOGENOUS INHIBITOR OF NITRIC OXIDE SYNTHASE, ASYMMETRIC DIMETHILARGININE (ADMA) INHIBITS FLOW DEPENDENT DILATION OF ISOLATED ARTERIOLES

J. Tóth[1], I. Wittmann[2], J. Nagy[2], A. Koller[1,3],
[1]Dept. of Pathophysiology, Semmelweis University, 1445-Budapest, Hungary, [2]2nd Dept. of Internal Medicine and Nephrology, University of Pécs, 7624-Pécs, Hungary and [3]Dept. of Physiology, New York Medical College, Valhalla, NY 10595, USA

The important signalling molecule, nitric oxide (NO) is produced by NO synthase (NOS) from L-arginine. Previous studies have shown that in metabolic diseases, such as hyperhomocysteinemia, diabetes mellitus and also in hypertension, liver and kidney diseases the serum level of ADMA - an endogenous inhibitor of NOS - increases, which may interfere with the regulation of vasomotor tone and activity. The direct effect of ADMA on the arteriolar function however, is not known. We hypothesized that ADMA inhibits NO mediation of flow-induced dilation of arterioles. Isolated arterioles from rat gracilis muscle (~150 μm at 80 mmHg) were treated with indomethacin, then incubated with ADMA (10^{-4} mol/L). ADMA decreased dilations to acethylcoline and completely eliminated dilations to increases in intraluminal flow (10-30 μL/min). Incubation of arterioles with the NOS substrate L-arginine (10^{-4} mol/l) restored flow-induced dilation. These effects of ADMA were similar to those of synthetic NOS inhibitor N^{ω}-nitro-L-arginine methyl ester (L-NAME 10^{-4} mol/l). We suggest that in various diseases the increased level of ADMA could interfere with NO mediation of flow-induced dilation, which could lead to increased microvascular tone and disturbed regulation of wall shear stress. Our findings may also explain the beneficial effect of L-arginine supplementation on vascular functions when serum level of ADMA is elevated. (Supported by Hungarian Nat. Sci. Res. Funds, OTKA T-034779, and T-043788 and NIH USA HL-46813)

OIR 7

VASOPRESSIN TREATMENT IN HEMORRHAGIC SHOCK

A.T. Cheung, B. Driessen, S. Ramanujam, M.A. Barbosa, D.M. Chan, V. Asfour, L. Zarucco, P. Burns, P.C. Chen, J.S. Jahr, and R.A. Gunther.
Departments of Pathology & Laboratory Medicine and Surgery, Univeristy of California, Davis School of Medicine, Davis, CA, 95616, U.S.A.

Vasopressin treatment, commonly used to redistribute blood flow and improve cardiac output (CO) in hemorrhagic shock, can lead to adverse effects as evidenced by occasional necrotic skin lesions and gastrointestinal varices. We hypothesize that these lesions may have resulted from severe reduction of blood flow caused by extensive post-vasopressin vasoconstriction. To test this hypothesis, computer-assisted intravital microscopy was used to study the real-time post-vasopressin microvascular changes in a canine severe hypovolemia model. The bulbar conjunctiva was used as a readily accessible non-invasive microvascular site in this study. Anesthetized mongrel dogs (n=9) were splenectomized and severely hemorrhaged (~50% blood loss) to induce hemorrhagic shock. Vasopressin was infused (n=6) as an IV loading bolus (0.4 IU/kg) followed by a 1-hr infusion (0.08 IU/kg/min). Dogs receiving an equal volume of saline (8.3 mL/kg) served as controls (n=3). Within minutes after vasopressin treatment, significant ($P<0.05$) decreases in venular diameter and changes in arteriole:venule ratio resulted. In addition, blood flow stopped in most (>95%) conjunctival vessels; in the few vessels which still maintained blood flow, the red-cell velocities were significantly ($P<0.05$) reduced. Some capillaries and small arterioles, which were visible before vasopressin treatment, disappeared from view. Post-vasopressin tissue oxygenation values decreased significantly ($P<0.05$), correlating with the changes in venular diameter and red-cell velocity. Paradoxically, there was no significant post-vasopressin improvement in CO. The ischemia arising from vasopressin treatment may explain the occurrences of necrotic lesions and gastrointestinal varicies in some shock patients

OAP 1

BLOOD FLOW DYNAMICS AND INTRAVASCULAR OXYGEN TENSION OF TUMOR MICROVESSELS UNDER PHOTODYNAMIC TREATMENT

H. Minamitani[1], N. Shibuya[1], Y. Iwata[1], A. Ushiyama[2], C. Ohkubo[2]
[1]Graduate School of Science & Technology, Keio University, Yokohama, 223-8522 Japan, [2]National Institute of Public Health, Shirogane, Tokyo, 108-8638 Japan

Photodynamic therapy (PDT) is accomplished by laser light excitation of photosensitizer accumulated in malignant tissue. The therapeutic effect is thought to involve direct tumor cell death as well as tumor vascular stasis. This study was designed to examine the effect of the photochemical reaction on angiogenesis and blood flow dynamics of tumor microcirculation. We developed an *in-vivo* microscopic technique to measure blood flow and oxygen tension (pO_2) simultaneously under PDT. The experiments were performed in male BALB/C mice (6~8 weeks old). A small piece of mouse mammary tumor was implanted in a dorsal skinfold chamber allowing observation of blood flow. For measurement of vessel diameter and RBC velocity, FITC-dx was injected into the tail vein for contrast enhancement of RBCs against plasma flow, and the fluorescent images were analyzed using a high speed camera and image processor. pO_2 in arterioles, veins and tumor vessels were determined by oxygen-dependent quenching of the phosphorescence decay technique. Pd-TCPP was used as the pO_2 probe and was excited by a Nd:YAG SH pulse laser (532nm). Compared to tumor free mice, mean values of vessel diameter and wall shear rate were found to be lower in tumor vessels, while vascular shut-down time in tumor vessels was shorter. The pO2 profile of tumor vessels and surrounding tissue was clearly different from that of the normal vascular bed. The results indicate that the high occurrence of vascular stasis was due to reduction of the wall shear rate in tortuous shaped vessels with an irregular intravascular surface and to different oxygen tension profiles. The *in-vivo* microscopic technique used in this study enabled us to clarify the relationship between angiogenesis and oxygen tension in tumor microvessels.

OAP 2

HIGH INTRALUMINAL PRESSURE UPREGULATES ARTERIAL NAD(P)H OXIDASE AND RENIN ANGIOTENSIN SYSTEM VIA PROTEIN KINASE C

A Koller, A Csiszár, Z Ungvári
Dept. of Pathophysiology, Semmelweis University, 1445 Budapest, Hungary
Dept. of Physiology, New York Medical College, Valhalla, NY 10595, USA

Clinical and experimental studies have shown that in many, if not all forms of hypertension - regardless of the underlying pathological mechanisms - are associated with oxidative stress. Thus, we aimed to test the hypothesis that chronic presence of high pressure, itself contributes to increased arterial O_2^- production in vivo. High blood pressure was induced in rats by abdominal aortic banding (Ab). Rats with Ab had elevated pressure in vessels proximal and normal pressure in vessels distal to the banding, yet both vascular beds were exposed to the same circulating factors. Compared to normotensive hind limb arteries (HLA), hypertensive forelimb arteries (FLA) exhibited impaired dilations to acetylcholine and the NO donor SNAP, responses, which were enhanced by superoxide dismutase (SOD). Also, there was an enhanced vascular production of O_2^- in FLA, which was reduced by SOD or NAD(P)H oxidase inhibitors or protein kinase C (PKC) inhibitors. Interestingly, in FLA but not in HLA the activity of angiotensin converting enzyme (ACE) was increased and the ACE inhibitor captopril reduced the increased production of O_2^-. In cultured isolated arteries of normotensive control rats presence of high intraluminal pressure (160 mmHg, for 24 h) significantly increased O_2^- production compared to vessels that were exposed to 80 mmHg This increased O_2^- was reduced by inhibitors of ACE and PKC. Thus we propose that in various forms of hypertension chronic presence of high pressure, itself elicits arterial oxidative stress via two pathways

OAP 3

CARDIOTONIC PILL® IMPROVES ISCHEMIA-REPERFUSION-INDUCED MICROCIRCULATORY DISTURBANCES IN RAT MESENTERY

J-Y Han, M Oda[2], H Suzuki, Y Akiba, H Nagata, S Miura[3], H Ishii, T Hibi.
Department of Internal Medicine, School of Medicine, Keio Universitokyo. Tokyo,160-8582 Japan.
[2]International University of Health & Welfare and Department of Internal Medicine,Sanno Hospital,
[3]The 2nd Department of Internal Medicine, National Defense Medical College, Saitama, Japan

Cardiotonic Pill® (CP), which consists of Danshen and Notoginseng, has clinically been used in China for the medical treatment of vascular diseases. We examined the effects of oral administration of CP, Danshen or Notoginseng on I/R-induced rat mesenteric microcirculatory injury. Under sodium pentobarbital anesthesia, the mesenteric microcirculation in the ileocecal portion of male Wistar rat was observed through an inverted-type intravital microscope with a CCD or SIT camera. I/R was conducted by a ligation of the mesenteric artery and vein for 10 min and a subsequent release of the blood flow occlusion. We measured the venular diameters, numbers of adherent leukocytes, FITC-albumin leakage, dihydrorhodamine 123 (DHR) fluorescence and mast cell degranulation, with or without CP, Danshen or Notoginseng (each 0.4g/kg) via an orogastric tube 1hr before I/R. I/R increased the number of adherent leukocytes, albumin leakage, DHR fluorescence and mast cell degranulation. CP attenuated these changes observed after I/R, Danshen reduced the number of adherent leukocytes, albumin leakage and DHR fluorescence but not mast cell degranulation, whereas Notoginseng reduced the number of adherent leukocytes ADHR fluorescence and mast cell degranulation, but not albumin leakage. The presant study suggests that Cardiotonic Pill® orally administered protects the microvascular endothelium through the inhibition of leukocyte-endothelium interaction and the reduction of oxidative stress from I/R-induced injury.

OAP 4

INTRAVITAL INVESTIGATION OF THE EFFECTS OF AN ANTI-VASCULAR AND AN ANTI-ANGIOGENIC AGENT ON TUMOUR MICROVASCULATURE

L.Lucas, C.Mitchell, V.Prise, S.Hill, K.Jiang, P.Barber, G.Soff, G.Tozer.
Gray Cancer Institute, Northwood, HA6 2JR, UK

Tumours require an intact microvascular network to grow and metastasise. Combretastatin A-4-P (CA-4-P), a tubulin-binding anti-vascular agent, causes acute shutdown of tumour vessels leading to necrosis of the tumour core, with the rim remaining viable. The anti-angiogenic agent Angiostatin$_{4.5}$ ($AS_{4.5}$) induces endothelial cell (EC) apoptosis, inhibits EC proliferation and migration, and slows tumour growth in mice.

Dorsal skin-fold window chambers were surgically implanted in SCID mice under Hypnorm/midazolam anaesthesia and a tumour fragment of either human colon adenocarcinoma (HT29) or endometrial adenocarcinoma (EA) transplanted into the chamber. After vascularisation, HT29 tumours were treated with CA-4-P (2 x 30mg/kg i.p. with a 2hr interval). In a separate experiment, mice with EA were treated for 10 consecutive days with $AS_{4.5}$ (2mg/kg/day s.c.), starting 24hr after surgery. Controls received vehicle-only. Before intravital imaging, mice were injected i.v. with fluorescently labelled erythrocytes. Video images of tumour microvasculature were captured using transmitted and fluorescent light at a range of objective magnifications (2.5x–20x) and blood flow (BF) through individual tumour vessels was calculated.

At 30 min after the first dose of CA-4-P in HT29 tumours, the BF decreased to 2.6±1.1% and at 4 hours BF was 6.2±2.2% of the initial value. The growth of EA tumours treated with $AS_{4.5}$ was significantly slower than controls. On the basis of these observations we will investigate the usefulness of $AS_{4.5}$ in blocking tumour recovery after CA-4-P treatment.

OAP 5

EFFECTS OF AN ANTI-ANGIOGENIC AGENT ON GROWING TUMOUR MICROVASCULATURE: AN INTRAVITAL INVESTIGATION.

L.Lucas, C.Mitchell, V.Prise, K.Jiang, P.Barber, G.Soff, G.Tozer.
Gray Cancer Institute, Northwood, HA6 2JR, UK

Tumours require an intact microvascular network to grow and metastasise. The anti-angiogenic agent Angiostatin$_{4.5}$ ($AS_{4.5}$) induces endothelial cell (EC) apoptosis, inhibits EC proliferation and migration, and slows tumour growth in mice. Here we report the first ever study of the effect of $AS_{4.5}$ on tumour vasculature in situ.

Dorsal skin-fold window chambers were surgically implanted in SCID mice under Hypnorm/midazolam anaesthesia and a tumour fragment of endometrial adenocarcinoma (EA) was transplanted into the chamber. At 24hr after surgery, mice were treated for 10 consecutive days with s.c. injections of $AS_{4.5}$(2mg/kg/day). Controls received vehicle only. Still images were captured on days 1 to 11 at a range of objective magnifications (2.5x–20x). Vascular morphometry was analysed using in-house developed computer software.

The growth rate of EA treated with $AS_{4.5}$ was significantly slower from days 6 to 11 than controls (156±13% and 282±46% of their initial area, respectively). During vascularization (days 6 to 8), treated tumours had fewer small calibre capillaries and greater interstitial distance (on day 7: treated, 83±29μm; control, 20±3μm) than controls. Average vessel diameter and length, density, tortuosity and fractal dimension were equivalent in both experimental groups during tumour vascularization.

These results indicate that this type of endometrial adenocarcinoma adapts quickly to its microenvironment and is highly dependent on its vascular compartment. Furthermore, $AS_{4.5}$ treatment causes small but measurable changes in the tumour vasculature in situ, leading to significant tumour growth inhibition.

OAP 6

ARTERIAL COLLATERAL FORMATION INFLUENCED BY CYCLOIDAL VIBRATION.

Prof. Dr P. Lievens. Vrije Univeriteit Brussel, Laarbeeklan 103, 1090 Brussel, Belgium.

This pilot in vivo study on mice aimed to determine whether non invasive cycloidal vibration would stimulate the formation of arterial collaterals. The non invasive application of cycloidal vibration is known to stimulate microcirculation and fluid dispersal in the skin. This study was approved by the University Ethical Commission and involved 115 mice.
115 mice underwent a microsurgical procedure on the abdominal skin. A main artery in the abdominal skin was sutured. The mice were then split into two groups a control group (n=60) and an experimental group (N= 55). The animals in the experimental group then received a daily treatment of cycloidal vibration therapy on the abdominal region on the location of the ligated artery for 20 minutes. The animals in the control group did not receive any treatment. After different time intervals (1 week, 2 weeks, 1 month, 2-3 months) 10 to 15 of the animals in both groups were inspected under microscope by in vivo examination for arterial collateral formation. Parameters studied, existence of arterial collaterals, collateral function and the existence of arterial anastomsis.

Results : In the control group no formation of collaterals was observed. In 22 cases anastomosis was observed with a clear arterial flow toward an opposite artery. In the experimental group, in 47 cases anastomosis was observed. In a total of 12 cases functional arterial collaterals were observed. These collaterals had a diameter of normal size and the arterial blood flow was totally restored.

Conclusion: The application of noninvasive cycloid vibration may have influenced the formation of arterial collaterals. Further investigations are proposed.

OAP 7

FIBRIN IS A POTENT STIMULUS OF ENDOTHELIAL MIGRATION.

M. Potter J.F. Dye C. Linge and R. Sanders
RAFT Institute, Mount Vernon Hospital, Northwood, London HA6 2RN UK

Angiogenic ingress is critical for the integration of tissue engineered scaffolds. Extracellular matrix signals regulate the morphology of human placental microvascular endothelial cells (HPMEC) independently of angiogenic growth factor stimulation, with collagen, but not laminin, eliciting a pro-angiogenic invasive phenotype (sprouting and migration responses). We hypothesised that fibrin may synergistically stimulate invasion into collagen-based scaffolds.

Human term placentae were used with consent to establish HPMEC cultures from chorionic villous capillary fragments. Confluent cultures on cytodex beads were suspended in extracellular matrix gels in minimum medium (MM) with or without angiogenic growth factors and were fixed at 96hr. For each condition images of 10 beads from triplicate wells were recorded from at least 3 cell isolates, and individual cell migration was measured by image analysis (SigmaScan) expressed relative to the collagen/MM control. Multiple comparisons were analysed by ANOVA and Tukey tests. Invasion was optimal in 0.75mg/ml collagen (200μm). Addition of VEGF modestly stimulated this (maximally 1.4x at 5ng/ml) and other angiogenic growth factors (bFGF, aFGF, IL8, TNF) gave similar stimulation, not exceeding 2x. Invasion into fibrin was greater than into collagen (maximally 6.9x at 1.3mg/ml). Collagen/fibrin admixtures gave less invasion with increasing proportions of collagen. No other matrix component tested (fibronectin, GAGs) was as potent as fibrin. Angiogenic growth factors attenuated invasion in fibrin/collagen gels. Analysis of proteolytic fibrin fragments has located a potent stimulatory domain.

We conclude that fibrin is a critical regulator of angiogenesis. It stimulates invasion in collagen gels and is more potent than VEGF or other extracellular matrix components.

Wednesday, 8th September
Plenary Symposium 1 - *Illusion of Reperfusion: Microvascular Integrity as the Key Factor in Successful Postischemic Reperfusuion*

1.1 Abstract not Available

1.2

THE ORIGINS OF THE MECHANISM FOR LEUKOCYTE RECRUITMENT/ACTIVATION IN A POSTISCHEMIC MICROCIRCULATION: APPLICATION TO SHOCK AND MULTIORGAN FAILURE

Geert W. Schmid-Schönbein
Department of Bioengineering, Whitaker Institute of Biomedical Engineering, University of California San Diego, La Jolla, CA 92093-0412, USA.

Physiological shock is accompanied by strong cell activation and inflammation. The inflammation affects virtually all cellular reactions in the microcirculation, and leads from mildly elevated permeability to cell apoptosis and organ failure. There is no understanding of the mechanisms that lead to inflammation. We propose a new hypothesis for the origin of humoral inflammatory mediators in shock. It was possible to trace the source of the inflammatory mediators to powerful digestive enzymes synthesized in the pancreas as part of normal digestion. Digestive enzymes have the ability to digest all biological tissues and are fully activated in the intestine. Self-digestion is prevented by compartmentalization within the mucosal epithelial barrier. Under conditions of intestinal ischemia or epithelial stimulation, however, the mucosal barrier becomes permeable to pancreatic enzymes allowing entry into the wall of the intestine. This process leads to self-digestion of intestinal extracellular matrix proteins and tissue cells and production of hydrophobic and hydrophilic small molecular weight inflammatory mediators. Inhibition of pancreatic enzymes in the lumen of the intestine serves to attenuate the inflammation in several forms of shock. Self-digestion by pancreatic enzymes may be a more universal mechanism for inflammation in the microcirculation.
(Supported by USPHS Grant HL 67825).

Thursday, 9th September
Plenary Lecture - *Microvascular Mechanisms for Inflammation and Organ Injury in Hypertension*

1.1

MICROVASCULAR MECHANISMS FOR INFLAMMATION AND ORGAN INJURY IN HYPERTENSION

Geert W. Schmid-Schönbein
Depart. Bioeng., Whitaker Institute of Biomedical Engineering, Univ. of Cal. San Diego, La Jolla, California 92093-0412, USA.

Hypertension is associated with genetic mechanisms that predisposes to an enhanced susceptibility as well as fully developed inflammatory reactions. The underlying mechanism for this propensity to inflammation is not well defined and it is uncertain how it is associated with the hallmark of hypertension, i.e. an elevated arterial blood pressure. In recent years, increasing evidence has been advanced in experimental and human hypertensives to suggest that excessive oxygen free radicals are produced in the circulation. Experimental forms of hypertension show that the free radical production is not only limited to the arterial side of the circulation but is equally prominent on the venous and venular side, vessels without an elevated blood pressure. In addition, there is evidence for a reduced nitric oxide formation, and enhanced apoptosis among cells of the microcirculation. In several forms of hypertension, endothelial apoptosis can be detected, which at the level of capillaries leads to loss of blood microvessels (rarefaction). In the spontaneously hypertensive rat, the oxygen free radical formation and apoptosis are driven by a glucocorticoid mechanism. Glucocorticoids cause a suppression of the leukocyte adhesion to endothelium, including P-selectin expression, while at the same time they serve to suppress the mechanical fluid shear stress response, an important anti-inflammatory mechanism. A key characteristic of hypertension is an increased susceptibility to secondary inflammatory mediators. The utility of anti-inflammatory interventions to reduce the complications in hypertension remain to be explored.
Supported by a grant from the USPHS HL10881.

Plenary Symposium 3 - *Clinical Microcirculation*

3.1

MICROVASCULAR CHANGES IN ALVEOLAR DISTRACTION OSTEOGENESIS

Lindeboom J.A.H.[1] and Mathura K.R.[2]
[1]Department of Oral and Maxillofacial Surgery
[2]Department of Physiology, Academic Medical Center, Amsterdam, The Netherlands

Distraction osteogenesis is an accepted treatment for the correction of bone deficiencies. The key of ossification is the vascular change into the callus because the osteogenesis follows after the angiogenesis. The purpose of this study was to describe vascular changes during alveolar distraction osteogenesis. Alveolar callus distraction was performed in 10 patients with alveolar ridge deficiencies. After a mucoperiosteal flap a horizontal osteotomy was made and placement of an alveolar distractor was performed. The distraction device was activated after 5 days of latency. The distraction protocol included a distraction rate of 1 mm a day. Microvascular images were obtained with the use of orthogonal polarization spectral (OPS) imaging. At day 1 postoperatively until the end of consolidation microvascular regeneration was assessed by monitoring of changes in capillary density.
All patients had a good response to the osseous distraction. No dehiscence or infections were observed. In all patients microvascular changes consisted of a decrease in capillary density and capillary index immediately after surgery to an increase in capillary density and capillary index during the early stages of distraction. During the consolidation phase capillary density and capillary index returned to preoperative levels.
Increase in vascular response mainly occurs in early stages of distraction.
OPS imaging provides images of sufficient quality to monitor, describe and assess the microvascular changes in distraction osteogenesis

3.2

THE MICROCIRCULATION IN CRITICAL ILLNESS.

E Christiaan Boerma[1,2], Peter HJ van der Voort[2], Can Ince[1].
[1]Department of Physiology, Academic Medical Centre, University of Amsterdam
[2]Department of Intensive Care, Medical Centre Leeuwarden, The Netherlands.

The treatment of shock remains an important clinical challenge in intensive care today. In hypovolemic obstructive and cardiogenic shock, hypotension occurs as a result of a decrease in cardiac output which results in altered tissue metabolism. In septic shock however hypotension occurs as a redistribution of volume caused by regional microcirculatory dysfunction in the presence of either normal or high cardiac output. Resuscitation from shock involves volume supplementation in combination with vasotonica, inotropics, corticosteroids and/or antibiotics aimed at correction of tissue perfusion and restoration of normal cellular metabolism. Particularly in septic shock however apparent adequate resuscitation based on correction of global hemodynamic and oxygen derived parameters is not per-se related to correction of regional dysoxia. The gut is considered as a particular sensitive organ in this respect due its sensitivity to dysoxia and the importance of maintaining its barrier function, and needs therefore to be monitored (1).
In our study we have investigated the behaviour of sub-lingual and intestinal microcirculation in critically ill septic patients during shock and resuscitation using OPS imaging (e.g.2,3). Measurements of the intestinal microcirculation was accomplished in critically ill patients with either ilea or colon stomas. Simultaneously we measured sub-lingual and mucosal villi microcirculation to investigate the microcirculatory response of these organs to sepsis. In this category of patients we found no correlation between the two microcirculatory beds. In some patients there was low to no flow in the intestines and normal microcirculatory flow sublingually, and in other patients we found the opposite. We also investigated the relation between peripheral temperature (as a surrogate for peripheral flow) and sublingual microcirculatory. Again we found no correlation between these two parameters.Our results are consistent with the idea that during sepsis there is a disparity in reaction of the different organ systems to hemodynamic failure. Analysis of the clinical progress of these patients in relation to their microcirculatory hemodynamics is expected to elucidate the role of microcirculatory failure in critically ill patients.

3.3

OPS-IMAGING: A NEW WAY TO OBSERVE THE MICROCIRCULATION.

Keshen R. Mathura, Can Ince
Department of Physiology, Academic Medical Center, University of Amsterdam, The Netherlands.

Orthogonal Polarization Spectral Imaging (OPS) makes use of green (540 ± 10 nm) polarized light to observe the microcirculation in living tissue. By using an orthogonally positioned polarizing filter in front of the CCD camera, the reflected light (which is still polarized) is filtered from the image. The light that has penetrated the tissue and has scattered for about 10 times before returning to the imaging system, has lost its polarization and is able to pass the orthogonal polarizer. The green light is absorbed by the hemoglobin in the erythrocytes. The end result of is a crisp image of black erythrocytes flowing thru the tissue. Because only scattered light is used for the final image, the light travels from the deeper layers of the tissue to the camera. This produces a back-lit effect of the final image where the light comes from deeper layers of the tissue illuminating the area of interest. OPS-imaging has evolved from application in large microscopes to a small handheld device that can easily be applied in patients and even during surgery. The first prototypes of these handheld devices used brightfield illumination. The images were clear, but superficial irregularities in the tissue were also clearly visible. The second generation prototype (which we use extensively today) uses darkfield illumination resulting in a clear and irregularity-free image. We first validated the technique by comparison to the golden standard in clinical microcirculation research, intravital capillary microscopy. (1) We were successful in imaging the microcirculation of the human brain during neurosurgery for the first time.(2) Consequently we used OPS-imaging to identify microcirculatory pathologies in brain tumors during surgery.(3) Finally we used sublingual OPS-imaging to monitor and evaluate the adequacy of resuscitation procedures in critically ill septic patients in the intensive care.(4)
OPS-imaging continues to be perfected and new modalities are being added and tested. We believe that OPS-imaging will become a new and easy to use bedside monitoring and diagnosis tool for doctors in the 21st century.

3.4

MICROCIRCULATORY SHUNTING DURING SHOCK AND RESUSCITATION.

Can Ince, Department of Physiology, Academic Medical Center, University of, Amsterdam, The Netherlands
e-mail: c.ince@amc.uva.nl

Whether tissue distress seen during sepsis is caused by tissue dysoxia (the condition where oxygen delivery to the tissues is insufficient to support mitochondrial respiration) or by cytopathic hypoxia (due to mitochondrial respiratory dysfunction ATP can no longer be synthesized despite adequate oxygen availability) is a source of debate (1-3). Clinically this controversy manifests itself as an explanation for the condition in sepsis and shock where despite correction of systemic oxygen delivery variables, regional dysoxia and a deficit in oxygen extraction persist. Our hypothesis has been that this condition is explained by the shunting of weak microcirculatory units in various organs (2,3). Here oxygen transport goes straight from the arterial to the venous compartment leaving the microcirculation hypoxic. That this is the case in shock and resuscitation we have demonstrated in hemorrhage, endotoxemia and anemia using the Pd porphyrin quenching of phosphorescence technique to measure microvascular pO2 (mpO2) in pig models of shock and resuscitations (e.g. 2-8). In these investigations we studied both the response of the mpO2 of the serosal and mucosal compartments of the porcine gut as well as that of the more vital organ such as the heart and kidney. We did this to investigate the regional variations between the different organ systems in response to resuscitation from sepsis as well as the response of the different compartments within one organ system (e.g. the gut). We knew from previous investigations that sepsis causes a dysfunction of autoregulation (9). We therefore hypothesized that during resuscitation the presence of an inflammatory component such as occurs during sepsis would result in more severe microcirculatory shunting either between the microcirculations of the different organ systems and/or between the different compartments within a single organ system. Indeed this turned out to be the case. Whereas fluid resuscitation from hemorrhagic shock (e.g. no inflammatory component) resulted in correction of both the serosal and mucosal mpO2, fluid resuscitation following septic shock (having the same depth of shock as in hemorrhage) was in the gut only affective in resuscitating the mucosal microcirculation. This resulted in a hypoxic serosa associated with elevated gastric CO2 (6). Based on the idea that active recruitment of the microcirculation is needed for adequate resuscitation from sepsis we hypothesized that vasodilator therapy can recruit microcirculatory units by increasing the microcirculatory forcing pressure (2,10). We found that NO donors improved microcirculatory oxygenation and oxygen extraction and also gastric pCO2 in a porcine model of sepsis (6). To apply these insights into the clinical treatment of septic shock we applied the OPS technique (e.g. 11,12) to directly observe sub-lingual microcirculation in septic shock patients. These results confirmed our animal studies where pressure guided resuscitation from septic shock resulted in shunting of the microcirculation with stasis in the capillaries but perfusion in the larger vessels (13). Resuscitation aimed at recruiting and opening the microcirculation by use vasodilatory therapy (nitroglycerine) as hypothesized from the animal studies described above, affectively restored microcirculatory perfusion in these septic patients (13). The recent finding that capillary perfusion deficit, but not values of systemic hemodynamic or oxygen derived parameter predicts death in septic shock patients has made microcirculatory monitoring of potential clinical importance in the treatment of septic patients (14,15).

Plenary Symposium 4 - *Critical Experimental Studies: A More Effective Way to Translate Basic Research Into Therapeutic Options?*

4.1

THE PROBLEM: COSTLY FAILURES OF CLINICAL STUDIES BASED ON PROMISING EXPERIMENTAL DATA.

D. Seiffge
Aventis Pharma, DG Thrombosis & Degenerative Joint Diseases, Industriepark Höchst, H 825, D-65926 Frankfurt-Main, Germany

In nearly all areas of intensive research with high clinical impact many promising concepts have and will be developed based on highly sophisticated experimental research. But, despite the large number of interesting therapeutic interventions that decrease damage or dysfunction in experimental animals, a high number of expensive clinical trials have produced negative results when testing the same agents in men!
Why is the outcome of corresponding clinical studies sometimes disappointing? How can we explain this discrepancy between bench and bedside studies? In this process a lot of personal enthusiasm and money may be consumed. In experimental research the problem exists that the definition of concepts and mechanisms is rated higher than effective development of therapeutic modalities (i.e. timing of treatment, age and associated illnesses, morphological and functional differences between the organs of humans and animals, mode of evaluation of efficacy, plasma concentration of drugs and side-effects, etc.). Despite the fact that concepts are based on presentation of potentially novel and effective approaches, negative preclinical results remain difficult to publish.
Existing baseline-risks for individual development phases are calculated using the so-called "New York Productivity Model", and show a probability to reach next milestone less than 50% in preclinical blocks, 25% in phase I/IIa, 80% in phase IIb/III of clinical development.
Can we establish valid risk assumptions on the basis of critical studies for individual subhurdles during different phases of development?

4.2

THE FACTS: THE ISCHAEMIA/REPERFUSION STORY AS AN EXAMPLE FOR FAILURES IN DEVELOPMENT OF PHARMACEUTICAL STRATEGIES

John M. Harlan, M.D.
Division of Hematology, University of Washington, Seattle, WA 98195

Ischemia-reperfusion (I/R) injury has been hypothesized to contribute to the pathology of diverse clinical disorders. Many investigators have demonstrated that blockade of leukocyte adhesion to endothelium affords striking protection in multiple animal models of I/R injury. Despite the encouraging pre-clinical results, clinical trials of leukocyte adhesion blockade in putative clinical I/R syndromes have been disappointing overall. There have been eight phase 2 or phase 3 trials of adhesion antagonists – three in myocardial infarction, three in stroke, and two in traumatic shock. None of the trials showed efficacy in meeting primary end-points.
There are a number of potential explanations for the failure of adhesion blockade in these clinical trials. First, the design of the some of the trials may not have been adequate to test the underlying hypothesis that leukocytes mediate a reperfusion injury. Second, it is possible that leukocytes are not a major mediator of clinical reperfusion injury. Other mediators, such as complement or oxidants, may be critical in the clinical setting. Finally, and perhaps most likely, the various animal models of I/R injury may not be valid models of human diseases. In the human disorders the ischemic injury may well be predominant and any component of reperfusion injury may not be significant enough to detect in clinical end-points. Having travelled from 'bench to clinic', it is now important to return to the bench to investigate the reasons for the failure in the clinic.

4.3

THE ANALYSIS: DEVELOPMENT OF NEW DRUGS: STRUCTURES, MECHANISMS, AND COSTS IN DIFFERENT PHASES

H.A.J. Struijker Boudier
Cardiovascular Research Institute Maastricht (CARIM), Dept. of Pharmacology and Toxicology, Universiteit Maastricht, P.O. Box 616, 6200 MD Maastricht, The Netherlands

Drug development is a highly complex and costly process. The average time of development is 10-12 years at a cost of close to 1 billion dollars. Basic research nowadays focuses on development of candidate drugs using molecular biological target discovery and chemical lead discovery and optimization. High-throughput technologies have increased the number of potential targets and lead compounds drastically. The next step in development is the profiling of series of compounds to a candidate drug using in vitro and in vivo model systems. After an average of 4 years, about 25% of the candidate drugs are taken into preclinical and 10% ultimately into clinical development. After another 6-8 years of development, less than 2% of the original candidate drugs is registered. The largest leap in costs and loss of candidate drugs is due to lack of sufficient therapeutic efficacy. This implies that a range of models rather than a single one should be used to assess therapeutic efficacy. After a period of speeding up target and lead discovery, there is now an urgent need to improve the process of therapeutic value assessment. The development of drugs against atherosclerosis will be used as an example to illustrate the various phases of drug development.

4.4

THE APPROACH: CRITICAL EXPERIMENTAL STUDIES

Axel R Pries
Dept. of Physiology, Charité CBF, Arnimallee 22, 14195 Berlin, Germany

The usual pathway for development of new parmacological treatment options starts from a ^theoretical concept or an empirical observation. Potential drugs are then investigated in simplified cell or animal models prior to the elaborate steps of clinical testing. In this process, the costs incurred at each development level increase by orders of magnitude. The aim of 'critical experimental studies' -inserted between the classical experimental studies and the clinical testing- is to reduce the probability of costly failures on the clinical level by stepping up efforts and discriminatory power of the experimental level. The experimental paradigm is shifted from 'proof of principle', hoping for positive results to 'only the best will survive' trying to filter out ineffective approaches. A number of parameters referring to animal models used in experimental studies which usually differ from the clinical situation have to be considered: homogeneous versus heterogeneous genetic background, optimal versus less well controlled administration, age, co-morbidity. Experiments taking into account these factors will require considerable efforts due to higher n-numbers, use of more species and genetically heterogeneous models, etc.. Also, the attitude of involved scientists and the respective publication pathways have to adapt to a scheme in which the production of 'failures' is as important as successful tests. However, the summed costs will still be only a fraction of one late dropout in clinical testing. Thus, the introduction of 'critical experimental studies' could make the overall process of drug development more effective and less costly and allow the development of a larger number of effective treatment options.

Thursday, 9th September

Parallel Symposium 1 - *Retinal Microcirculation: Experimental and Clinical Aspects*

1.1 Abstract not available

1.2

VASCULAR RISKS IN AMD

Professor Alon Harris

Age related macular degeneration (AMD) is the leading cause of irreversible visual loss in the United States, responsible for an estimated 1.2 million cases of severe visual loss. Several theories of pathogenesis have been proposed including primary RPE senescence, genetic defects such as ABCR gene mutations (which encodes a retinal rod photoreceptor), and primary ocular perfusion abnormalities.

Although the theory of RPE senescence is appealing, it does not fully account for the wide variety of clinical presentations in AMD, including various forms of drusen, hyperpigmentation, and RPE atrophy in nonexudative AMD as well as CNVM formation in exudative AMD. Another pathogenic theory, consequently, involves primary vascular changes in the choroid which then secondarily affect the RPE and lead to AMD; specifically, it is theorized that lipid deposition in sclera and Bruch's membrane leads to impaired choroidal perfusion, which would in turn adversely affect metabolic transport function of the retinal pigment epithelium.

With regard to the role of choroidal perfusion defects, it is well known that the choriocapillaris supplies the metabolic needs of the retinal pigment epithelium and the outer retina; a primary perfusion defect in the choriocapillaris could account for some of the physiologic and pathologic changes in AMD. Some authors have suggested that delayed choroidal filling may correlate with diffuse thickening of Bruch's membrane. Eyes with delayed choroidal filling angiographically have been shown to harbor discrete areas of increased threshold on static perimetry. Delayed choroidal filling has been noted angiographically in patients with exudative ARMD and there is some evidence that choroidal blood flow is abnormal in patients with nonexudative AMD.

In summary, there appears to be a specific derangement in the choroidal circulation in patients with AMD. Vascular defects have been identified in both nonexudative and exudative AMD patients using fluorescein angiographic methods, laser Doppler flowmetry, indocyanine green angiography, and color Doppler imaging. Although these studies lends some support to the vascular pathogenesis of AMD, it is not possible to determine if the choroidal perfusion abnormalities play a causative role in nonexudative AMD, if they are simply an association with another primary alteration, such as a primary RPE defect or a genetic defect at the photoreceptor level, or if they are more strongly associated with one particular form of this heterogeneous disease.

Thursday, 9th September

Parallel Symposium 2 - *Red Blood Cell Interaction with Blood Vessel Wall Endothelium in Circulatory Disorders*

2.2

MULTIFACTORIAL NATURE OF SICKLE RED CELL ADHESION TO VASCULAR ENDOTHELIUM

Dhananjay K. Kaul
Department of Medicine, Albert Einstein College of Medicine, 1300 Morris Park Avenue, Bronx, N.Y. 10461, U.S.A.

The defining feature of sickle cell anemia is periodic occurrence of painful vasoocclusive crisis. Although the painful vasoocclusive crisis could not propagate without red cell sickling, the emerging evidence indicates that initial events may involve a complex interplay of multiple factors. Factors that promote trapping and sickling of red cells in the microcirculation are likley to trigger vasoocclusion. Among the potential factors, the increased propensity of sickle red cell adhesion to vascular endothelium may play a significant role in the initiation of a vasoocclusive episode. Studies with ex vivo and sickle transgenic models have shown that sickle red cells adhere exclusively to venular endothelium. Multiple factors and adhesion molecules may participate in this interaction. Unlike leukocyte-endothelium interactions in which rolling, firm adhesion and extravasation of leukocytes occur in a sequential fashion via reasonably well-defined receptor-ligand interactions, sickle red cell adhesion follows no such paradigm. We propose that sickle red cell adhesion is multifactorial in nature. A host of modulating factors (i.e., red cell heterogeneity and deformability) and receptor-ligand interactions may participate in this interaction. Using an ex vivo microvascular preparation, we show an important role of sickle red cell heterogeneity, certain adhesion molecules (e.g., von Willebrand factor, thrombospondin and alpha V beta 3 intergin) and inflammatory stimuli in this interaction. Thus, multifactorial nature of sickle red cell adhesion needs to be considered in designing antiadhesive threrapy in vivo.

2.5

MEMBRANE COMPONENTS IN THE INTERACTION OF RED BLOOD CELLS WITH ENDOTHELIAL CELLS.

Koshkaryev Alexander, Barshtein Gregory and Yedgar Saul.
Biochemistry Department, The Faculty of Medicine, The Hebrew University, P.O.B. 12272 Jerusalem 91120, Israel.

Summary
Under normal flow-induced shear stress RBCs adherence to EC is insignificant. However, in pathological conditions that are associated with damaged RBC properties, RBC adhesiveness is determined by the biochemical components of their membrane, and changes in these factors in pathological conditions are responsible for altering RBC/EC interaction. The present study was undertaken to identify RBC intrinsic membrane components that determine their interaction with EC. Results: 1) Both band-3 clustering and translocation of phosphatidylserine (PS) to RBC surface induce enhanced RBC adherence. 2) Treatment of RBC with band-3 aggregating factor very effectively induced translocation of PS to the cell surface, suggesting an interrelation between these processes. Conclusion: Band-3 clustering and PS translocation are the key membrane factors in RBC/EC interaction. The interdependence and the cause-and-effect relation between them has yet to be studied

3.1 Abstract not available

3.2

NEW MICROSCOPIC TECHNIQUES: ONE APPROACH FITS ALL?

D.W. Slaaf[1,2], M.A.M.J. van Zandvoort[1]
[1]Department of Biophysics, University Maastricht, and [2]Department of Biomedical Engineering, Eindhoven University of Technology
PO Box 616, 6200 MD Maastricht, the Netherlands

In classical intravital studies, usually bright field and/or fluorescence microscopy are used. The numerical apertures of objective and condenser, and the setting of the condenser diaphragm determine resolution. The considerable depth of field makes detection possible of flowing [or rolling] blood cells within the microvessels. The disturbing influence of over- and underlying structures is a disadvantage. Removal of such structures may be accomplished by deconvolution techniques. With the use of confocal microscopy, thin optical sections are obtained, which can be used for 3-D reconstruction. In vivo, however, preparations are often moving due to heartbeat and respiration, and cells may move out of the optical section.

Processes as atherosclerosis manifests itself in larger vessels where a high penetration depth is required. The overlying tissue has a detrimental effect on image quality, even in the case of confocal microscopy. This may be overcome by using two-photon excitation fluorescence microscopy. The usually red excitation light is less sensitive to scattering and excitation occurs only in a thin plane about focus. It should be noted, however, that the resolution in two-photon microcopy is less, because it is solely determined by the wavelength of the excitation light. A considerable advantage of two-photon microscopy is that it can easily be combined with assessment of fluorescence lifetime, which provides another mechanism for contrast or concentration or activity of molecules.

Many optical microscopy methods are available varying from relatively cheap to very expensive. Depending on the research question to be answered, various techniques may be required. A simple solution that suits all is not available.

3.3

TWO-PHOTON MICROSCOPY AND ITS APPLICATION TO IMAGING INSIDE MOUSE ATHEROSCLEROTIC ARTERIES.

Marc A.M.J. van Zandvoort, Dick W. Slaaf
Department of Biophysics, University Maastricht, Universiteitssingel 50, 6229 ER Maastricht, the Netherlands

Two-photon microscopy combines the advantages of traditional fluorescence microscopy (high contrast and sensitivity) and confocal fluorescence imaging (high resolution, 3D reconstruction) with increased penetration depth and reduced photodamage in dense tissues. It thus enables long term *in vivo* imaging in many biological tissues.

In the past years two-photon microscopy has developed from a technical innovation into a technique that has found various applications in biomedical research, such as tumor angiogenesis and brain functionality.

After an introduction to the concept of two-photon microscopy and its main characteristics, in this presentation focus is on its possible role in atherosclerosis research. First, results on histological slices of atherosclerotic mouse arteries are compared with traditional imaging to illustrate its contrast capabilities. Second, data on intact carotid arteries are presented and it is noted that for these experiments two-photon microscopy is a prerequisite. Finally, we show images and movies of *in vivo* imaging of arteries in atherosclerotic mice. Various subjects of interest, such as the imaging of apoptosis, angiogenesis, NO metabolism and 3D structures will be discussed.

3.4

TWO PHOTON IMAGING AND NEUROVASCULAR COUPLING IN THE RAT OLFACTORY BULB: QUANTITATIVE ANALYSIS OF THE RELATIONSHIP BETWEEN CHANGES IN NEURONAL ACTIVITY AND CHANGES IN CAPILLARY RED BLOOD CELL FLOW.

E. Chaigneau, F. Debarbieux, M. Oheim, E. Audinat, S. Charpak.
Inserm U603, ESPCI, 10 rue vauquelin, Paris, France

Analysis of the spatio-temporal coupling between neuronal activity and cerebral blood flow requires the precise measurement of the dynamics of red blood cell (RBC) flow in individual capillaries that irrigate activated neurons. We have recently used two-photon microscopy *in vivo* to image individual RBCs in glomerular capillaries in the rat dorsal olfactory bulb (Chaigneau et al., PNAS 2003). We found that odor stimulation evokes capillary vascular responses which share the main properties of neuronal responses: they are odorant- and glomerulus-specific, and precisely outline the region of synaptic activation. Because a glomerulus contains a single type of olfactory bulb output cells, the mitral cells, it should be possible to correlate odor-evoked changes in RBC flow with the firing of mitral cells as long as their activity can be monitored simultaneously. Recently, we have shown that each action potential fired by mitral cells backpropagates to the glomerulus where it is detected as a transient increase in $[Ca^{2+}]_i$ (Debarbieux et al, J. Neurosci. 2003). Because each glomerulus contains less than 50 output cells which tend to fire synchronously, we are investigating, using two-photon microscopy imaging of both RBC capillary flow and neuronal activity, the quantitative relationship between the number of action potentials fired by mitral cells and the resulting change in glomerular RBC flow that occur during odor stimulation.

5.1

GAP JUNCTIONS AND ENDOTHELIUM-DEPENDENT HYPERPOLARIZATION

T.M. GRIFFITH
Department of Diagnostic Radiology, Wales Heart Research Institute, University of Wales College of Medicine, Cardiff, UK CF14 4XN

There is growing evidence that electrotonic mechanisms underpin the NO-independent EDHF-type relaxations that are observed in many artery types following administration of endothelium-dependent agonists or SERCA inhibitors such as cyclopiazonic acid (CPA). Such responses can be attenuated by synthetic inhibitory peptides targeted against the Gap 26 and 27 domains of the extracellular loops of the major vascular connexins (Cxs 37, 40 and 43). These peptides do not affect endothelial hyperpolarization directly, but interrupt its electrotonic spread into and through the media via myoendothelial and homocellular smooth muscle gap junctions. Endothelial stimulation by agonists or CPA also evokes a prostanoid-independent increase in endothelial and smooth muscle cAMP synthesis/accumulation. This cyclic nucleotide may enhance gap junctional communication by promoting connexin phosphorylation via protein kinase A and/or recruitment of connexin proteins to the cell membrane, and thus play a central role in the EDHF phenomenon. Indeed, P site inhibitors of adenylyl cyclase such as dideoxyadenosine abolish the ability of myoendothelial gap junctions to allow the spread of endothelial hyperpolarization into the media of rabbit arteries with corresponding loss of relaxation, a finding that can be reversed by inhibiting cAMP hydrolysis with the phosphodiesterase inhibitor IBMX. Under control conditions IBMX also enhances electrotonic signalling within the media by increasing smooth muscle cAMP levels, and thereby potentiates EDHF-type relaxations. These findings highlight a previously unrecognized degree of complexity in NO-independent vascular signalling.

5. 2

NITRIC OXIDE AND REGULATION OF GAP JUNCTIONS.

Ulrich Pohl and P. Kameritsch, University of Munich (LMU), Germany.

Gap junctions (GJ) are clusters of channels that allow transfer of low molecular weight substances and electrical currents between neighbouring cells. In the vascular system these channels are formed by various combinations of the connexins (Cx) 37, 40, 43 and 45. GJ allow the signal exchange within endothelial and smooth muscle layer and, in addition, between both cell layers. Moreover, recent data indicate that transmigration of leukocytes can be altered significantly by precedent gap junctional coupling with endothelial cells. Though our understanding of the coupling between endothelial cells and smooth muscle cells or leukocytes is still incomplete it is obvious that the transfer of signals via GJ can be regulated. Recent experiments suggest that the endothelial autacoid NO plays a specific role in this regulalion. NO is decreasing the conductivity for small charged molecules such as cyclic nucleotides, calcium or IP3 of gap junctions. There is, however, also some evidence that NO, under certain conditions, can improve coupling by increasing the formation of new gap junctions. Experiments in transfected HeLa-cells reveal that this different action of NO is based on selective effects on different connexins. NO increases the membrane incorporation of Cx40-GJ and reduces the permeability of already incorporated GJ formed by Cx37. These data suggest that the coupling between the vascular cells is subject to modulation by endothelial derived compounds. The functional significance of this modulation for vasomotor responses and vascular growth is not yet fully understood and subject of further investigations.

5.3

CONDUCTED VASODILATATION

C. de Wit
Physiologisches Institut, Universität Lübeck, Ratzeburger Allee 160, 23538 Lübeck, Germany

Intercellular communication along the vessel may contribute to the coordination of arteriolar behaviour within the microcirculation. This is especially important under conditions of high flow due to downstream vasodilatation because upstream vessels would limit flow increases under these circumstances. Only with a concomitant upstream dilatation maximal flow increases can be achieved. Communication along the vessel is reflected by the conduction of vasodilatations along the arterioles after locally confined application of endothelial stimulator substances (e.g. acetylcholine or bradykinin). The vasodilatation is initiated by a locally induced hyperpolarization in endothelial and smooth muscle cells that spreads along the cells of the vascular wall through intercellular channels, called gap junctions. They are composed of connexins that form low resistance channels providing the pathway for the spread of locally initiated electrical signals along the vessel. In vascular cells different connexin proteins are expressed (Cx40, Cx43, Cx37, and Cx45), of which Cx40 is especially important for the conduction of vasodilatations as conducted responses are attenuated in Cx40-deficient animals. Interestingly, these mice are hypertensive suggesting that intercellular communication through this connexin contributes to the control of peripheral vascular resistance. Since Cx40 is mainly expressed in endothelial cells, the endothelial layer seems to provide the main pathway for signal transduction along the vessel. In fact, it has been demonstrated that the disruption of the endothelial cell layer in a confined area along the arteriole abrogates signal transmission along the vessel and eliminates conducted vasodilatations upstream of this injured site.

5.4

BIOCHEMICAL CHARACTERIZATION OF EPOXYEICOSATRIENOIC ACIDS AS MORE THAN ENDOTHELIUM-DERIVED HYPERPOLARIZING FACTORS

I. Fleming
Institut für Kardiovaskuläre Physiologie, Johann Wolfgang Goethe-Universität, Theodor Stern Kai 7, 60590 Frankfurt am Main, Germany

Cytochrome P450-derived epoxyeicosatrienoic acids (EETS) have been suggested to act as an endothelium-derived hyperpolarizing factor (EDHF) as they are able to activate Ca^{2+}-dependent K^+ channels and thus to elicit the hyperpolarisation and relaxation of vascular smooth muscle cells. Although initially assumed to be generated within endothelial cells but to act mainly on vascular smooth muscle cells, EETs are now thought to elicit the majority of their effects within the cells of origin. Indeed, the first step in any EDHF-mediated response is an endothelial cell hyperpolarisation and recent data indicate that EETs play a central role in the regulation of this response. EETs modulate endothelial cell hyperpolarisation, not by directly affecting the activity of Ca^{2+}-dependent K^+ channels but rather by affecting Ca^{2+} influx via the TrpV4 channel. EETs are also now known to have a number of additional intracellular targets and to play an active role in the regulation of gene expression and vascular homeostasis that is not necessarily linked to their effects on membrane potential. In endothelial cells EETs activate adenylyl cyclase to increase the generation of cyclic AMP and activity of protein kinase A and thus transiently increase communication through gap junctions. The same signalling cascade also results in the activation of the cyclic AMP-response element-binding protein (CREB) and an increase in the expression of COX-2. This latter effect contributes to the angiogenic effects of EETs which also involves the transactivation of the epidermal growth factor receptor and matrix metalloproteases as well as endothelial cell migration.

Plenary Symposium 6 - *Programming of Vascular Dysfunction*

6.1

FETOPLACENTAL VASCULAR FUNCTION IN DIABETIC PREGNANCY

J. Coleman & C. Hillier
Department of Medicine and Therapeutics, Ninewells Hospital, University of Dundee. DD1 9SY Scotland, UK

Pregnant women with diabetes have an increased risk of stillbirth and pre-eclampsia through mechanisms associated with dysfunction of the fetoplacental vasculature. Adrenomedullin (ADM) and endothelin-1 (ET-1) are thought to be important mediators of fetoplacental vascular function and both vasoactive factors have been implicated in the pathophysiology of diabetes. This study describes the loss of ADM vasodilation and the loss of protective ET_B signalling in the fetoplacental vasculature of mothers with type 1 diabetes mellitus and suggests mechanisms of action.

Isolated stem villous arteries from healthy and type 1 diabetic mothers were mounted on a pressure myograph. Concentration response curves were constructed to ADM (following preconstruction with U46619, 10nM) and ET-1. In control mothers, dilation to ADM was attenuated by L-NAME, ODQ and SQ22536 but not indomethacin or charybdotoxin and apamin ($p<0.01$). ADM vasodilation was significantly augmented by zaprinast and milrinone ($p<0.05$). The villi from diabetic mothers showed a dramatic decrease in vasodilation. BQ788 caused significant augmentation of vasoconstriction to ET-1 ($p<0.05$). Arteries from diabetic mothers showed a dramatic vasoconstriction more than double that of controls ($p<0.001$). BQ788 had no effect on diabetic arteries. Comparison of stem villous mRNA using RT-PCR showed an increase in Receptor Activity Modifying Protein1 (RAMP1) expression in villi from diabetic mothers and a significant decrease in ET_B receptor expression. A similar alteration in RAMP1 and ET_B mRNA expression was seen in human placental cells grown in high glucose.

Vasodilation is decreased in diabetes due to upregulated RAMP1 expression and a loss of protective ET_B signalling caused by high glucose.

6.2

FETAL ENDOTHELIAL DEVELOPMENT AND FETAL VASCULAR CONTROL

E Villamor, K Ruijtenbeek, CGA Kessels, JGR De Mey, CE Blanco.
Departments of Pediatrics and Pharmacology, Research Institute Growth and Development (GROW), University of Maastricht, The Netherlands.

Birth weight is the resultant of intrauterine growth, which is mainly determined by the availability of nutrients and oxygen to the fetus. When this availability is reduced, fetal protective adaptations will be initiated. These adaptations may persistently affect organ function and structure, leading to pathology at later stages of life. Many studies have focused on fetal malnutrition as a cause of cardiovascular disease in later life. However, the most common cause of intrauterine growth retardation is placental insufficiency, which is a combination of both malnutrition and chronic hypoxia.

Loss of the modulatory role of the endothelium may be a critical and initiating factor in the development of systemic and pulmonary hypertension. Hypoxia-induced alterations of endothelial properties have been demonstrated in fetal systemic and pulmonary arteries. The chicken embryo is a suitable model for studying the effects of adverse conditions, such as hypoxia and malnutrition, without the direct interference of maternal (endocrine, metabolic and cardiovascular) factors.

We have demonstrated in the chicken embryo that chronic exposure to moderate hypoxia, leading to growth retardation, increases arterial sympathetic innervation and reduces endothelial vasodilator function at embryonic day 19. In contrast, prenatal hypoxia transiently reduced pulmonary arterial contractile reactivity but did not affect endothelial function of pulmonary arteries and did not induce structural remodeling of the pulmonary vascular bed.

6.3

PROGRAMMING THE ENDOTHELIUM DYSFUNCTION IN UTERO: ROLE OF SUPEROXIDE ANION, NITRIC OXIDE AND ANGIOTENSIN II.

Franco MCP, Akamine EH, Fortes ZB, Tostes RCA, Carvalho MHC, Nigro D.
Department of Pharmacology, University of São Paulo, Brazil.

It is well known that intrauterine undernutrition (IU) contributes to the development of cardiovascular disease in adulthood. In addition, the vascular diseases that have been linked to IU are characterized by endothelial dysfunction. The aim of this study was to explore the mechanisms involved in programming of endothelium dysfunction in utero. Female pregnant Wistar rats were fed either normal or 50% of the normal intake diets, during the whole gestational period. In male offspring, arteriolar diameter was measured in vivo by intravital microscopy before and after application of bradykinin (BK) or acetylcholine (ACh) in the absence or presence of SOD mimetic, tetrahydrobiopterin (BH_4) (NOS cofactor) or apocynin (NADPH-oxidase inhibitor). Superoxide anion generation (hydroethidine method) was studied in the absence or presence of apocynin, BH_4 or losartan. Arterial blood pressure, NOS and SOD activities, NO production (DAF-2), angiotensin II (ANGII) concentration (HPLC) and AT_1, $p22^{phox}$, $gp91^{phox}$ and eNOS gene expression (RT-PCR) were determined. IU induced hypertension, decreased vasodilation to ACh and BK. Topical application of SOD mimetic, apocynin and BH_4 *significantly improved the altered arteriolar responses to ACh and BK. Decreased SOD and NOS activities, reduction in NO production, increased superoxide concentration, enhanced local ANGII concentration, attenuation of oxidative stress by* BH_4, *apocynin and losartan and improvement of NO production after treatment with* BH_4 *were observed. IU did not alter the gene expression for eNOS,* AT_1, $p22^{phox}$ *and* $gp91^{phox}$.

This study shows that IU programmed endothelium dysfunction by: 1) enhancing oxidative stress, which is associated with decreased SOD activity and increased activation of NADPH oxidase via ANGII-mediated mechanism; 2) decreasing NO production by impairment of BH_4 *pathways.activity and increased activation of NADPH oxidase via ANGII-mediated mechanism; 2) decreasing NO production by impairment of* BH_4 *pathways.*

6.4

CLINICAL IMPLICATIONS OF ENDOTHELIAL DYSFUNCTION IN LOW BIRTH WEIGHT SUBJECTS

M Norman
Department of Women and Child Health, Karolinska Institute, S-182 88, Stockholm, Sweden

Systemic dysfunction of the vascular endothelium precedes hypertension, cardiovascular disease and NIDDM. Already as neonates, subjects with low birth weight (LBW) exhibit endothelial dysfunction that persists into childhood and adult life. The prevalence of endothelial dysfunction among healthy young subjects may be an expression of early disease susceptibility and this could be an important link in understanding epidemiological associations between LBW and increased risk of cardiovascular disease in adults. The highest risk for endothelial dysfunction has been found in thin babies born at term whereas endothelial function seems to be preserved after preterm birth. In addition, studies in birth weight discordant monozygous twins indicate that endothelial dysfunction associated with LBW does not have a pure genetic origin. Taken together, these findings point at the third trimester during pregnancy as a sensitive period during which fetal growth failure may adversely affect vascular development.

There are several clinical implications. First, LBW should be added to the list of risk factors predicting cardiovascular disease. Second, factors that are known to damage the vascular endothelium and that have the potential to be modified during pregnancy should be targeted, aiming at intervention. Such factors include fetomaternal levels of homocysteine and blood lipids, oxidative stress and inflammation. Third, long-term outcomes should be included in the discussion of optimal timing for delivery of a growth retarded fetus. Finally, in those born too small and too early, there are accumulating data that nutrition, growth and stress also after birth are important for later cardiovascular function, structure and regulation.

6.5

TRANSGENERATIONAL PROGRAMMING OF ENDOTHELIAL FUNCTION.

C. Torrens, L. Poston* and M.A. Hanson
Centre for Developmental Origins of Health & Disease, University of Southampton, SO16 5YA, UK. *Maternal & Fetal Research Unit, GKT Medical School, London, SE1 7EH, UK.

In the rat dietary protein restriction during pregnancy results in raised blood pressure, endothelial dysfunction and impaired glucose handling in the offspring. Maternal blood pressure is associated with that of the offspring while impaired endothelial function in the pregnant offspring of protein restricted dams may mediate transgenerational inheritance. In contrast inheritance down the male lineage may suggest a genomic mechanism, such as epigenetic modifications. Wistar rats were fed either a control (C; 18% casein) or protein restricted diet (PR; 9% casein) throughout pregnancy. When mature, F_1 male and female offspring were mated with control animals to produce male (Cm & PRm) and female (Cf & PRf) lineage. Systolic blood pressure (SBP) of F_2 offspring was assessed by tail cuff plethysmography and vascular function of small mesenteric arteries by wire myography. In PRf F_2 offspring SBP was raised compared to Cf. SBP was also higher in male F_2 offspring from PRm compared to Cm, but not different between female PRm and Cm. Vasoconstriction to phenylephrine (PE) was enhanced while vasodilatation to ACh was impaired in male PRf compared Cf rats. In male PRm F_2 offspring, vasoconstriction to PE was attenuated and vasodilatation to ACh increased compared to the Cm group. This data demonstrates that cardiovascular risk factors can be transmitted to the F_2 offspring of protein restricted rat dams. The different effects seen in the male and female lineages suggest that such transgenerational transmission may be mediated by different mechanisms from each parent.
This work was supported by the BHF.

6.1

E-SELECTIN AND CXCR2-DEPENDENT NEUTROPHIL ARREST DURING INFLAMMATION

Klaus Ley, Michael L. Smith, Timothy S. Olson, Cardiovascular Research Center and Dept. of Biomedical Engineering and Molecular Physiology, University of Virginia, Charlottesville, VA, 22908, USA

During inflammation, leukocytes cells roll along the walls of postcapillary venules and eventually are arrested upon activation by surface-bound chemokines. Arrest chemokines have been identified for naïve T and B lymphocytes as well as monocytes, but not for neutrophils. Unlike monocytes and lymphocytes, rolling neutrophils systematically slow down before arrest (Kunkel E.J. et al., J. Immunol. 164: 3301, 2000). In vitro assays suggest that both E-selectin and chemokines can trigger arrest of rolling neutrophils, but E-selectin$^{-/-}$ mice have normal levels of adherent neutrophils in inflamed venules, castimg doubt on the importance of this mechanism. To test whether chemokine-induced neutrophil arrest in vivo can be unmasked by blocking E-selectin, we investigated neutrophil adhesion in inflamed cremaster muscle venules in TNF-α-treated CXCR2$^{-/-}$ or wild-type (WT) mice injected with E-selectin blocking mAb 9A9. To block chemokine receptor signaling through Gαi, we treated E-selectin$^{-/-}$ or WT mice with pertussis toxin (PTx) i.v. Neutrophil adhesion was similar to that found in WT mice in CXCR2$^{-/-}$, E-selectin$^{-/-}$, PTx-treated WT, or mAb 9A9-treated WT mice, demonstrating that neither E-selectin nor Gαi signaling were required for arrest. However, TNF-α-induced neutrophil adhesion was completely abrogated in E-selectin$^{-/-}$ mice treated with PTx and significantly reduced in CXCR2$^{-/-}$ mice treated with the E-selectin blocking mAb. In thioglycollate-induced peritonitis, PTx treatment blocked neutrophil recruitment into the peritoneum of E-selectin$^{-/-}$ mice, but had only a minor effect in WT animals. These data show that E-selectin- and chemokine-mediated arrest mechanisms are overlapping in this model of inflammation and identify CXCR2 as an important neutrophil arrest chemokine receptor in vivo.

Supported by National Institutes of Health grants EB 02185 and HL54136 to K.L.

6.2

COMPARATIVE ANALYSIS OF T LYMPHOCYTE INTERACTION WITH MICROVESSELS IN THE CEREBRAL CORTEX AND THE SPINAL CORD *IN VIVO*

Mohammad Farhadi[1], Melanie Laschinger[2], Peter Vajkoczy[1], Britta Engelhardt[2,3]
[1]Department of Neurosurgery, Clinic Mannheim, University of Heidelberg, Germany; [2]Max-Planck Institute for Molecular biomedicine, Münster, Germany, [3]Theodor-Kocher Institute, University of Bern, Switzerland

Employing a novel spinal cord window preparation which allows to directly visualize central nervous system (CNS) white matter microcirculation by intravital fluorescence videomicroscopy we demonstrated before that T cell interaction with the CNS white matter microvasculature is unique due to the lack of T cell rolling and that α4-integrin mediates the G-protein independent capture and subsequently the G-protein dependent adhesion strengthening of T cell blasts to microvascular VCAM-1. We have now compared these observations to T lymphoblast interaction with cerebral cortex and pial microvessels by employing a cranial window preparation which allows to directly visualize pial and cortical microvasculature by intravital fluorescence videomicroscopy. Although microhemodynamics in the cerebral cortex were found to differ from the CNS white matter T cells were found to interact with cerebral cortex microvessels in a similar manner as obesrved in spinal cord microvessels before. Differences in the angioarchitecture of cerebral cortex and spinal cord microvessels and differences in the molecular mechanisms involved in T cell interaction in both vascular beds will be discussed.

Employing a novel spinal cord window preparation which allows to directly visualize central nervous system (CNS) white matter microcirculation by intravital fluorescence videomicroscopy we demonstrated before that T cell interaction with the CNS white matter microvasculature is unique due to the lack of T cell rolling and that α4-integrin mediates the G-protein independent capture and subsequently the G-protein dependent adhesion strengthening of T cell blasts to microvascular VCAM-1. We have now compared these observations to T lymphoblast interaction with cerebral cortex and pial microvessels by employing a cranial window preparation which allows to directly visualize pial and cortical microvasculature by intravital fluorescence videomicroscopy. Although microhemodynamics in the cerebral cortex were found to differ from the CNS white matter T cells were found to interact with cerebral cortex microvessels in a similar manner as obesrved in spinal cord microvessels before. Differences in the angioarchitecture of cerebral cortex and spinal cord microvessels and differences in the molecular mechanisms involved in T cell interaction in both vascular beds will be discussed.

6.3

INAPPROPRIATE LEUKOCYTE ACTIVATION IN VASCULITIS AND DISSEMINATED INTRAVASCULAR COAGULATION.

keith Norman, University of Sheffield, UK

Ordered presentation of chemoattractants and adhesion molecules permits circulating leukocytes to efficiently target tissues where there is injury, infection or perceived risk. Leukocytes first attach to and subsequently roll along vascular endothelium, are activated by chemoattractants, firmly adhere and finally are attracted into tissues where they target specific locations. Although this multistep paradigm for leukocyte recruitment allows precise control throughout, the system is not flawless, and can be misled. The presence of bacteria (or their products) in the blood, for example, invokes a vigorous inflammatory response that can throw the innate immune system into chaos.

We have used intravital microscopy of the mouse cremaster muscle to investigate consequences of inappropriate (intravascular) leukocyte activation induced on a background of pre-existing inflammation. RB6-8C5 antibody, which depletes neutrophils in unstimulated mice, caused leukocyte activation, arrest of the cremaster microcirculation, microvascular injury and death in TNFα-primed mice. Genetic deficiency, antibody blockade or pharmacological inhibition of selectins protected animals from this reaction. Complement-depletion was also strongly protective. In more recent studies using LPS in place of RB6-8C5 we have measured more localised reactions associated with leukocyte and platelet aggregation as well as petechial haemorrhage. These LPS-induced responses are both complement and TLR4-dependent.

6.4

L-SELECTIN LIGAND FUNCTION IN SIALYLTRANSFERASE ST3GAL-IV DEFICIENT MICE.

M.Sperandio[1], M.Smith[3], T.Olson[3], L.Ellies[4], O.Linderkamp[1], R.Nobiling[2], J.Marth[5], and K.Ley[3]
[1]Children's Hospital and [2]Dept. of Experimental Surgery, University of Heidelberg, Germany, [3]Cardiovascular Research Center, University of Virginia, Charlottesville, USA, [4]Cancer Center and [5]Department of Cellular and Molecular Medicine, University of California, La Jolla, USA.

L-selectin is expressed on most leukocytes and mediates leukocyte rolling in inflamed microvessels and high endothelial venules (HEV) by binding to L-selectin ligands. Previous studies using sialidase treatment suggested a role of terminal sialic acid residues for L-selectin ligand function in vivo. To investigate the role of the sialyltransferase ST3Gal-IV on L-selectin ligand function in vivo, we compared leukocyte rolling in venules of untreated and TNFα-treated cremaster muscles and in Peyer's patch HEV of ST3Gal-IV deficient mice and littermate control mice. In cremaster muscle venules, treatment with blocking mAbs against P- and E-selectin almost completely abolished L-selectin mediated rolling in ST3Gal-IV$^{-/-}$ mice, but not in littermate control mice, suggesting that L-selectin ligand function is dependent on ST3Gal-IV in this setting. In contrast, leukocyte rolling in Peyer's patch HEV was not significantly different between ST3Gal-IV$^{-/-}$ and control mice, suggesting that L-selectin ligands on Peyer's patch HEV are mostly independent of ST3Gal-IV. Our data show that L-selectin ligands relevant for rolling in inflamed microvessels of the cremaster muscle are completely dependent on ST3Gal-IV, while L-selectin ligands in Peyer's patch HEV are not affected by the absence of ST3Gal-IV.

6.5

INVOLVEMENT OF THE TYROSINE KINASE SYK IN THE CONTROL OF LEUKOCYTE POLARIZATION

J. Schymeinsky and B. Walzog
Dept. of Physiology, Ludwig-Maximilians-Universität, 80336 Munich, Germany.

The tyrosine kinase Syk, which is associated with the β-subunit of the β_2 integrins (CD11/CD18), is activated upon β_2 integrin-mediated adhesion. Here, we elucidated the role of Syk for b2 integrin-mediated leukocyte functions using neutrophil-like differentiated HL-60 cells and the monocytic cell line THP-1. By means of confocal microscopy, we detected a homogenous distribution of Syk in unstimulated HL-60 cells in suspension. In contrast, stimulation of HL-60 cells with the bacteria-derived chemoattractant f-Met-Leu-Phe (fMLP, 100 nM) in the presence of immobilized fibrinogen showed an enrichment of Syk at the lamellipodium forming site where Syk colocalized with F-actin in the adherent and polarized cell. This finding was confirmed using THP-1 cells stimulated with the monocyte chemoattractant protein-1 (MCP-1, 10 ng/ml). In contrast, no enrichment of Syk at the lamellipodium was detectable in fMLP-stimulated HL-60 cells in suspension indicating that the redistribution of Syk depended on β_2 integrin-mediated adhesion. Treatment of HL-60 cells with the Syk inhibitor piceatannol (30 μM) abolished the redistribution of Syk suggesting that the redistribution required Syk activation. However, the inhibition of Syk did not impair adhesion but it led to an excessive formation of lamellipodia in activated HL-60 cells and thereby interfered with ordered cell polarization. This finding suggests a role for Syk in the stabilization of the bipolar phenotype, a prerequisite for chemotactic migration which is critical for efficient recruitment of leukocytes to sites of inflammation. (Supported by DFG WA 1048/2-1)

7.1

DEVELOPMENT AND PRINCIPLE OF THE SERVONULLING TECHNIQUE IN CAPILLARY PRESSURE MEASUREMENTS.

D.W.Slaaf
Department of Biophysics, University Maastricht, PO Box 616, 6200 MD Maastricht, the Netherlands

Knowledge of the pressure distribution in microvessels is important for our understanding of perfusion of the microvasculature and transcapillary movement. The first micropressure measurements were performed with the Landis technique (1930). A micropipette was used to cannulate single capillary loops in human skin. Movement of red blood cells into the cannula was used to counterbalance the pressure in the microvessel with the pressure in the connected manometer. The frequency response of such a system is very low: no information is obtained about pressure pulsatility. This method has also been extended to tissue pressure measurement, where movement of an air bubble was used to assess pressure differences.

Micropipettes are generally used to record trans-membrane potentials in excitable cells. In 1964, Curt Wiederhielm understood that resistance of a pipette would change when blood, with a relatively high electrical resistance compared to the KCl solution inside the pipette, would enter the pipette. He developed the servonulling micropressure measurement technique. A micropipette was hydraulically connected to a bellows pump, which generated the backpressure required to keep the electrical resistance of the pipette constant. The frequency response is up to more than 30Hz, if the compliance of the system (tubing) is low and air bubbles are avoided. Coupling between the fluid of the pipette and the pressure generating part of the system may also be accomplished by air. In such a system, however, it is important that large volumes of air can be rapidly displaced. Air bubbles still have to be avoided in the hydraulic part of the system.

The micropressure technique requires expert experimental skills. It has been successfully applied to animal as well as to human studies.

7.2

WHAT INFORMATION ABOUT MICROCIRCULATORY PHYSIOLOGY HAS BEEN GAINED FROM CAPILLARY PRESSURE MEASUREMENTS.

C.C.Michel, Biomedical Sciences, Imperial College, London, SW7 2AZ UK.

A rapid expansion of microcirculatory physiology followed the description of the servo-nul micropipet technique by Wiederhielm for measuring microvascular pressure, P_c, (Am.J.Physiol. 1964; 207:173-176) and the introduction of other direct quantitative methods in the1970's. Flow-pressure relations were now investigated in single microvessels and the pre and post-capillary regulatory mechanisms were observed directly. Also new insights were gained of blood-tissue fluid exchange. Measurements of P_c in glomerular capillaries revised understanding of glomerular filtration and its regulation. At a more fundamental level, direct measurements of P_c undermined the textbook portrayal of Starling's Hypothesis of fluid filtering from the arterial end of capillaries and being absorbed at the venous end. When compared with plasma oncotic pressure and interstitial hydrostatic and oncotic pressures, direct measurements of P_c are inconsistent with this picture (Levick. Exp. Physiol. 1991; 76: 855-857). The picture is also inconsistent with the basic principles of fluid exchange where permeability to macromolecules is finite (Michel & Phillips. J.Physiol. 1987;388: 421-435) and this, coupled with lymph flow data, has revised views on how blood-tissue fluid balance is achieved (Michel. Exp.Physiol.1997; 82: 1-30). In the past few years, new models of microvascular fluid exchange) have been developed (Hu & Weinbaum. Microvasc.Res.1998; 58: 281-304) and new experiments (Hu et al. Am.J.Physiol.2000; 279: H1724-H1736; Adamson et al. J.Physiol. 2004, in press) have been carried out to test them. These continuing developments can all be seen as a consequence of direct measurements of P_c, many of which have been made on humans.

7.4

WHAT CAN WE LEARN FROM CAPILLARY BLOOD PRESSURES IN PATIENTS WITH LEG ISCHAEMIA?

J.C. de Graaff[1], D.Th. Ubbink[2]
Dept. of Anaesthesiology[1], St. Antonius Hospital, PO Box 2500, 3430EM Nieuwegein; Dept. of Vascular Surgery[2], Academic Medical Center, Amsterdam, The Netherlands.

Capillary perfusion and transmural pressure are delicately regulated by microvascular constriction mechanisms, which are activated upon a change in posture. Capillary flow is known to be disturbed in patients with severe peripheral arterial disease. To date, however, the influence of this disease on capillary pressure is unknown.

Systolic capillary pressure (CP, mm Hg) in the nail fold of the hallux and systolic toe blood pressure (TP, mm Hg) was measured in the sitting and supine positions in 8 patients with intermittent claudication (F2), in 7 patients with rest pain and/or ulcers (F3-4), and in 12 age-matched healthy controls (F0). For this purpose a capillary in the eponychium of the hallux was punctured under microscopic guidance using a micropipette, which was connected to a servo-nulling system.

TP and CP in the three groups were significantly ($p<0.001$) higher in the sitting than in the supine position. TP decreased significantly with increasing disease severity, but CP was comparable among the groups.

Sitting:	F0	F2	F3/4	p*	Supine: F0	F2	F3-4	p*
TP	140	104	64	<.01	91	49	14	<.01
CP	64	63	62	.19	22	23	16	.5

* Kruskal-Wallis test, to analyse differences between groups

AN INCREASE IN ORTHOSTATIC PRESSURE INCREASES BOTH TOE AND CAPILLARY PRESSURES. ARTERIAL INSUFFICIENCY OF THE LEG SEEMS TO LEAVE THE CAPILLARY PRESSURE UNSCATHED. LOCAL ARTERIOLAR VASOCONSTRICTION MECHANISMS APPEAR TO PLAY AN IMPORTANT ROLE IN THE DELICATE REGULATION OF CAPILLARY PRESSURE

7.5

THE RELEVANCE OF PRESSURE MEASUREMENTS IN LYMPHATIC CAPILLARIES

B.R. Amann-Vesti, MD
Angiology Division, University Hospital Zurich, Switzerland

The lymphatics comprise a one-way transport system for fluid and proteins by collecting them from the interstitial space returning them to the blood circulation. The technique of fluorescence microlymphography allows the visualization of the lymphatic capillaries of the skin in vivo and has provided the basis for studying the physiology and pathophysiology of the initial lymphatic system in vivo in humans. By using the servo-nulling technique intralymphatic pressure measurements had been performed in different forms of edema. In normal subjects intralymphatic pressure was 4.0±4.5 mmHg at the lower leg and 7.9±3.4 mmHg at the foot dorsum. In patients with lymphedema of the lower leg microlymphatic hypertension is present (15.0±5.1 mmHg).

Lymphatic contractility plays a crucial role in the regulation and generation of lymph transport. It has been shown that human lymphatic contractility can be influenced by a number of neural and humoral factors. By measuring intralymphatic pressure we have demonstrated that prostaglandin-F2-alfa reduced intralymphatic pressure in patients with lymphedema. A similar reduction had been measured after intensive physical treatment in these patients.

Pressure measurements in lymphatic capillaries in humans have provided important insights into the physiology of the lymphatic system. However, further studies on the regulation of human lymph transport are needed to provide better information for the treatment and prevention of lymphatic diseases.

10.2

CIRCULATING PROGENITOR CELLS: MOLECULAR MECHANISMS AND CLINICAL RELEVANCE

Christopher Heeschen, M.D.; J.W. Goethe University, Molecular Cardiology, Frankfurt, Germany

Recent studies demonstrated that postnatal neovascularization does not exclusively rely on sprouting of pre-existing vessels ("angiogenesis"), but involves bone marrow-derived circulating endothelial progenitor cells (EPCs). EPCs can be ex vivo--expanded out of isolated mononuclear cells or can be obtained by cultivation of $CD34^+$- or $CD133^+$-positive hematopoietic progenitors. Importantly, transplantation of EPCs was shown to promote postnatal neovascularization of ischemic tissue after myocardial infarction.[1]These experimental data suggest that circulating EPCs may contribute to improvement of neovascularization. Therefore, we investigated the regulation of EPCs in patients with coronary artery disease (CAD).

In a pilot trial (TOPCARE-AMI), we have investigated the safety and efficacy of intracoronary infusion of autologous bone marrow-derived or blood-derived progenitor cells (EPCs) for regeneration enhancement in patients with ischemic heart disease.[2]Meanwhile, more than 100 patients were randomly treated with mononuclear cells from bone marrow (BMC), which were isolated from bone marrow aspirates (50 ml) by gradient centrifugation (n=47), or blood derived progenitor cells (EPCs), which were ex vivo expanded for 3 days out of 250 ml peripheral blood in the presence of statins (n=53). There were no signs of an inflammatory response and no malignant arrhythmias suggesting that transplantation of progenitor cells appears to be feasible and safe. Statistically analyzed 4-month follow-up data are currently available for 58 patients with acute myocardial infarction (29 patients with BMC and 29 patients with EPCs). These data were compared to a matched, but non-randomized control group (n=15). Transplantation of progenitor cells was associated with significantly increased LV ejection fraction, improved regional wall motion, and reduced endsystolic LV volumes at 4-months follow-up. Coronary flow reserve in the infarct artery was normalized in BMC- and EPC-treated patients. Myocardial viability in the infarct zone as determined by PET was significantly increased at follow-up. There was no difference between EPC- and BMC-treated patients. Thus, transplantation of progenitor cells appears to be feasible and safe in the first 100 patients studied. Intracoronary infusion of bone-marrow-derived cells or circulating blood-derived cells may beneficially affect post-in-farction re modeling processes. To provide definitive evidence for the functional improvements after cell therapy, a randomized, placebo-controlled multicenter trial (REPAIR-AMI) has been started in April 2004.Importantly, circulating progenitor cells from patients with established CAD exhibit an impaired functional and migratory activity. The reduction of EPCs was correlated with risk factors for CAD such as hypercholesterolemia or age.[3,4]Consistent with the fact that nitric oxide (NO) plays an important role in neovascularization and NO bioavailability is typically reduced in patients with ICMP, we were able to demonstrate that the impaired neovascularization in mice lacking endothelial nitric oxide synthase (*Nos3*) is related to a failure of progenitor cell function and mobilization. [5] *Nos3*$^{-/-}$ mice show reduced vascular endothelial growth factor-induced mobilization of endothelial progenitor cells and increased mortality after myelosuppression. Intravenous wild-type progenitor cell infusion, but not bone marrow transplantation rescued the defective neovascularization of *Nos3*$^{-/-}$ mice in a model of hind limb ischemia implicating that progenitor mobilization from the bone marrow is impaired in *Nos3*$^{-/-}$ mice. Mechanistically, matrix metalloproteinase MMP-9, which is required for stem cell mobilization, was reduced in bone marrow of *Nos3*$^{-/-}$ mice. These findings demonstrate that Nos3, expressed by bone marrow stromal cells, critically influences recruitment of stem and progenitor cells, which may contribute to impaired regeneration processes in patients with ischemic heart disease, who are characterized by a reduced systemic NO bioactivity. Indeed, bone marrow stem and progenitor cells from patients with ischemic heart disease demonstrate a markedly reduced migratory response to stromal cell-derived factor-1. This may also limit their therapeutic potential for clinical cell therapy, especially when using an intravascular route of administration which requires the progenitor cells to extravasate against a chemoattractant gradient in order to invade and home to ischemic tissue. Monitoring the migratory and colony forming activity of stem/progenitor cells prior to cell therapy may serve as a surrogate test for identifying patients that may derive greater benefit from cell therapy. Indeed, a recent subanalysis of the TOPCARE-AMI trial revealed that the migratory capacity of the infused cells determines the functional improvement of the treated patients. [6]On the other hand, a recent experimental study suggests that fully functional bone marrow-derived EPCs from healthy donor mice restore the senescent host cardiac angiogenesis in a murine model of impaired neovascularization.[7]Thus, it is tempting to speculate that pharmacological or genetic manipulation of the functionally impaired BM-MNCs prior to reinfusion may improve their functional activity and, subsequently, may improve the patients' therapeutic benefit from cell therapy.

10.3

ADVANCES AND CHALLENGES IN ANTI-ANGIOGENIC AND TUMOR VASCULATURE TARGETED THERAPIES

Grietje Molema, Dept. Pathology and Laboratory Medicine, Medical Biology section, Groningen Institute for Drug Exploration (GUIDE), Groningen, Netherlands

New insights in the cellular control of tumor growth unveiled an essential role for tumor blood vessels in tumor mass progression, and identified tumor endothelial cells as an attractive target for therapeutic intervention. By their active involvement in neovascularization processes, tumor endothelium can be discriminated from non-diseased endothelium elsewhere in the body. Intracellular signal transduction pathways in tumor endothelium are spatiotemporally controlled to direct gene expression towards an angiogenic profile. A variety of small chemical entities and biotech based therapeutics have been developed to counteract this pro-angiogenic signalling and gene expression control. Moreover, tumor endothelial make-up of growth factor receptors and adhesion molecules is different from non-tumor endothelial cells. This makes them particularly attractive for vascular drug targeting approaches that aim at selective delivery of drugs / genes / effector cells (in)to the tumor endothelium, to interfere with tumor blood flow and induce tumor cell death. An overview will be given on the classes of drugs developed to inhibit tumor growth associated angiogenesis and their reported effectiveness. Furthermore, successful strategies explored to deliver effector systems selectively in tumor endothelium will be discussed. Focus will be on delivery systems for gene therapy and immunotherapy that obtain their specificity from (small molecule) homing ligands that specifically bind to epitopes overexpressed on pro-angiogenic tumor endothelial cells.

Pre-clinical studies on tumor vascular endothelium specific therapies showed strong anti-tumor effects. One of the reasons for lack of success in clinical studies is our poor understanding of tumor endothelial cell activation status in patients that should guide the choice of anti-vascular therapies. In animal tumor models, neovascularization stages are synchronised as a result of rapid outgrowth of tumors. Consequently, (targeted) drugs will attack the majority of vessels in the growing tumor. In cancer patients, however, tumor neovascularization stages are highly heterogenic. Only a fraction of the tumor endothelium will therefore be affected by a particular class of drug. By applying the newest technologies available, the molecular basis for heterogeneity in tumor endothelial cell behaviour in their pathological context are unravelled. By this means, we will learn to understand the reasons for failure and success of tumor vasculature directed therapies and identify new targets for (targeted) therapeutic intervention of angiogenesis driven diseases.

Saturday, 11th September
Parallel Symposium 11 - *From Endothelial Dysfunction to Atherothrombosis*

11.2

NO AS A MARKER OF ENDOTHELIAL DYSFUNCTION: CLINICAL CORRELATIONS

Carlota Saldanha
Instituto de Biopatologia Vascular, Faculdade de Medicina de Lisboa

Nitric oxide (NO) is a coproduct generated in the endothelial cell during the conversion of L- arginine on L-citruline by nitric oxide synthase (eNOS).

NO has an inhibitory action on cytokine induced expression of adhesion molecules and on cytokine production among others autocrine functions. As a consequence a pro inflammatory state will be unfavourable under normal physiological conditions.

However when NO bioactivity decreased at a dysfunctional endothelium cytokines could induced a procoagulant activity on the hemostatic system and different sorts of vascular diseases could be developed. For example genetic manipulation of eNOS in knockout mice results in hypertension and atherosclerosis.

Vasodilatory response to acetylcholine (ACh) by peripheral or coronary artery is a marker of endothelial function and its decreased predictive of cardiovascular events. The endothelial injury with loss of ACh dependent vasodilatation occurs in hypertension, diabetes and dyslipidemia which could be associated either to reduced NO production or increased release of reactive oxygen species.

11.3

OXIDATIVE STRESS AND INFLAMMATION MODULATE VASCULAR FUNCTION IN HYPERHOMOCYSTEINEMIA (HHCY)

A Koller, A Csiszar, Z Ungvari
Department of Pathophysiology, Semmelweis University, Budapest H-1445, Hungary
Department of Physiology, New York Medical College, Valhalla, NY 10595, USA

Elevated levels of homocysteine have been shown to be an independent risk factor for the development of coronary, cerebral and peripheral vascular diseases. Homocysteine is formed during the metabolism of the essential amino acid, methionine. The normal plasma concentration of Hcy ranges between 10-15 μmol/L and can increase due to genetic alterations and/or vitamin deficiencies affecting enzymes participating in the metabolism of homocysteine and methionine. We aimed to document the early changes in the function of microvessels in HHcy and reveal the underlying cellular and molecular mechanisms. In the early phase of experimental HHcy in rats we have found that flow dependent dilation of vessels is impaired due to endothelial dysfunction, whereas the dilator functions of smooth muscle remain unaffected. Endothelial dysfunction seems to be primarily to decreased bioavailability of nitric oxide (NO) and enhanced production of constrictor prostaglandins. These alterations are elicited by enhanced production of reactive oxygen species by NAD(P)H oxidase and/or xanthine oxidase. Oxidative stress in the presence of NO is known to result in an enhanced production of peroxynitrite. The oxidative and nitrosative stress observed in HHcy can promote the development of vascular inflammation, as indicated by the increased expression of inducible NO synthase, and TNFα. These pathophysiological processes may promote not only vascular dysfunction but also deposition of lipids in the vessel wall favoring the development of atherosclerosis.

(Supported by NIH 43023, 48613 USA and NSRF T-034779 Hungary)